The Complementary Formulary

Other books by the same author

Homoeopathy for Physicians
The Dental Prescriber
Die homöopathische Verordnung in der zahnärtzlichen Praxis
The Biochemic Handbook
Handbuch der homöopathischen Gewebesalze
The Traveller's Prescriber
The Infinitesimal Dose
A Textbook of Dental Homoeopathy*
The World Travellers' Manual of Homoeopathy*
Homöpathisches Reisehandbuch
Handboek Homeopathie voor de Wereldreiziger
Homoeopathic Remedies - An International Handbook

**shortly also available in Japanese*

Senior commissioning editor: Heidi Allen
Development editor: Robert Edwards
Production controller: Anthony Read
Desk editor: Jackie Holding
Cover design: Fred Rose

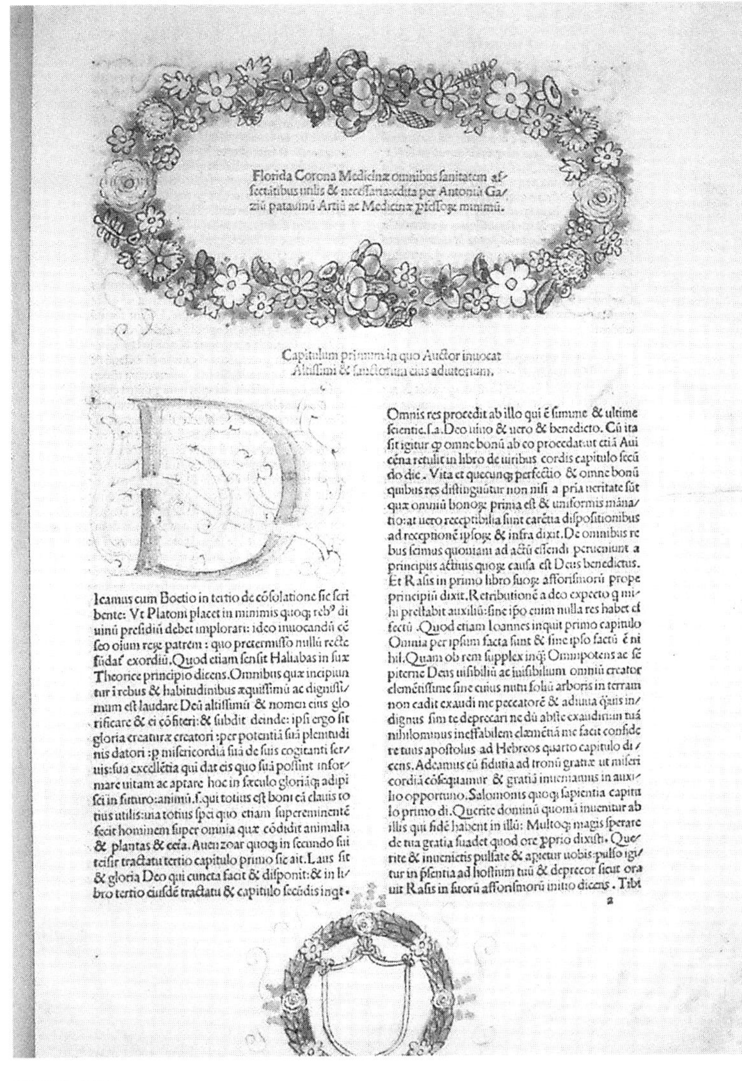

Frontispiece
Gazio, Antonio (*c.* 1463–*c.* 1520). Title page of *Florida Corona Medicinae* (The Floral Crown of the Art of Healing), printed in Venice by John & Gregory de Forlivio, 1491, 1st edition, Folio (31.3 × 22cm), 126 leaves. One of the earliest printed works on nutrition, dietetics and the conservation of good health. Gazio is said to have been physician to King Sigismund of Poland. However, he travelled a great deal, acquiring fame and wealth. For some time he lived in Hungary, but spent his last years at Padova in Italy.

The Complementary Formulary

A Guide for Prescribers

Dr Colin B Lessell

MB, BS (Lond), BDS (Lond), MRCS (Eng), LRCP (Lond), FBHomDA, DDFHom, HonFHMA

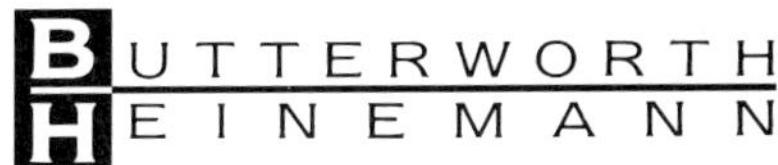

OXFORD AUCKLAND BOSTON JOHANNESBURG MELBOURNE NEW DELHI

Butterworth-Heinemann
Linacre House, Jordan Hill, Oxford OX2 8DP
225 Wildwood Avenue, Woburn, MA 01801-2041
A division of Reed Educational and Professional Publishing Ltd

 A member of the Reed Elsevier plc group

First published 2001

British Library Cataloguing in Publication Data
A catalogue record for this book is available from the British Library

Library of Congress Cataloguing in Publication Data
A catalogue record for this book is available from the Library of Congress

ISBN 0 7506 5389 2

www.bh.com

Composition by Scribe Design, Gillingham, Kent, UK
Printed and bound by MPG Books Ltd, Bodmin, Cornwall

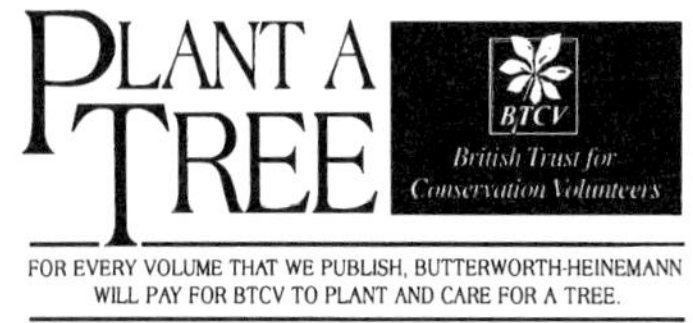

Contents

Quotation ix

Acknowledgements x

Disclaimer x

Introduction xi

Part 1 Quick Guide
A Quick Guide to the Use of the Formulary 3
An example from the text 8
Table of abbreviations 9
Table of Anglo-American spelling conversion 10

Part 2 General information
Section 1: Nutritional Supplements 13
Section 2: Herbal Medicines 16
Section 3: Homoeopathic Remedies 20
Section 4: Bach Flower Remedies 45

Part 3 The Formulary
The icons of the Formulary 51
The Formulary 53

Part 4 Additional Information
Appendix 1: Clinical manifestations and indications of some important syndromes 223
❑ Chronic gastrointestinal candidiasis 223
❑ Fibromyalgia 224

❑ Hypoglycaemia (non-diabetic/reactive) 224
❑ Iron deficiency 225
❑ Menopausal arthritis 225
❑ Reversible adrenal depletion 226
Appendix 2: Herb/drug/supplement interactions, side-effects and contraindications 227
Appendix 3: A new physics of homoeopathic pharmacy 233
Appendix 4: List of professional suppliers (with international mail order facilities) 255
Appendix 5: Index of medicaments 257
Nutritional supplements 257
Herbal medicines 260
Homoeopathic remedies 263
Bach Flower remedies 269
Injections 274
Ruta graveolens 274
Vitamin B_{12} (hydroxocobalamin) 274

OPINIONUM COMMENTA DELET DIES,
NATURÆ JUDICIA CONFIRMAT

*TIME EFFACES THE FABRICATIONS OF OPINION
BUT CONFIRMS THE JUDGMENTS OF NATURE*

CICERO (106-43 B.C.)

Acknowledgements

In the preparation of this text for professionals, I have had the advantage of consulting my colleague, Malcolm Fairbrother, MPS, of Bedford; and must thank him for his helpful advice on a large number of pertinent pharmaceutical matters; so, similarly, with regard to herbal issues, the semi-anonymous Melissa and Dawn of Phyto Products Limited of Mansfield. Additionally, I must thank Messrs. C. W. Daniel of Saffron Walden for allowing liberal use of material of mine previously published by them, especially *A Textbook of Dental Homoeopathy* and *The World Travellers' Manual of Homoeopathy*. Lastly, but not least, I must extend my appreciation to Heidi Allen, Commissioning Editor, Medical Books Division, of Butterworth-Heinemann. Undoubtedly, she gave me great encouragement in my labours by sharing and fostering my own enthusiasm for the project, whilst providing numerous editorial words of wisdom in good Oxford English.

Disclaimer

This book is intended only for the use of the properly qualified and registered health professional and the registered dispensing pharmacist. Whilst every effort has been made on the part of the author to convey everything as properly as possible, neither he, nor the publisher, shall accept responsibility for any inaccuracies, errors or omissions; nor for any untoward side-effects, undesirable medicinal interactions, other unfortunate results of therapy, or failures of treatment which result, might have resulted, or appear to have resulted, from the use of this book by either those duly qualified persons for whom it is intended or others.

Introduction

This book has been especially written for the professional prescriber and the dispensing pharmacist. Rather than being an unpractical, complex and voluminous textbook of complementary therapies, it is a highly select and pointed extraction from personal experience, current practice and literature. As such, it is designed for speedy and effective prescribing in busy clinical and OTC (over-the-counter) situations, which prevail in many complementary clinics, retail pharmacies and general medical practices throughout the world. Whereas the main topics of the book concern nutritional supplementation, herbal (botanic) prescriptions, homoeopathy and the Bach Flower Remedies, the practitioner or pharmacist must feel free to mingle other aspects of medicine with any propositions of my own. Should he or she be concerned about any adverse interactions with orthodox drugs, a glance at the table of Appendix 2 (in Part Four) should help to resolve the matter in less than one minute of precious time.

There is little doubt in my own mind, as is the case with many other health professionals, that the way forward in medicine is the adoption of more liberal, yet discerning, attitudes. It is a fact of life that many patients derive much benefit from a careful blend or medley of a variety of therapeutic techniques, both orthodox and unorthodox. One does not preclude the use of the other. Indeed, with the passage of time and the passing of antipathy, the unconventional often becomes the norm, as the history of pharmacy and medicine has so often elegantly displayed. I am sure that we are all aware of the increasing interest and demands of the public in the direction of the complementary therapies, and that at least a little of our work should be devoted to understanding and, perhaps, even practising them. To these ends, you should find that this book both clarifies and expedites a seemingly, at first sight, difficult task.

For convenience, the text is actually divided into four Parts. The most important for most readers, and by far the largest of the four, is Part Three, **The Formulary** proper, concerning prescriptions for particular diseases or syndromes, and arranged alphabetically. Those who are in a hurry to proceed should go immediately to Part One and read **A Quick Guide to the Use of the Formulary**, before turning to **The Formulary** proper. The details given there, albeit concisely, should be quite adequate to get you started on the right footing.

Those of a more cautious, stoical or analytical bent, however, should begin with Part Two, which contains much useful detail about the methodology and application of the main complementary disciplines which form the substance of this book. Here, there are four Sections. Section 1 is mainly devoted to *nutritional supplementation*, though with some comments on nutritional therapy in general; Section 2 to *herbal medicine*; Section 3 to *homoeopathy*; and Section 4 to *Bach Flower Remedies*. Having read these, proceed to the **Quick Guide to the Use of the Formulary**.

Part Four comprises five Appendices. Appendix 1 describes a number of important clinical syndromes with which the reader may not be familiar (such as chronic gastrointestinal candidiasis). Appendix 2, concerning herb/drug/supplement interactions, side-effects and contraindications, has already been mentioned, and will be valuable to most. Appendix 3 contains a new theory of the *physics of homoeopathy*, and should be of particular interest to many pharmacists. However, it does require a reasonable fundamental familiarity with homoeopathy and its pharmaceutical practices, and, where such knowledge is absent, it is wise to first read Section 3 of Part Two. Appendix 4 is merely a useful list of professional suppliers of the various medicaments (and reference books) described in the text. They are not of much use if you do not know where to get them, and many are easily mailed worldwide. Appendix 5 is an index of those medicaments, so that their various uses are more easily determined.

Throughout, I have assumed that the reader has a sound basic knowledge of general medicine, though not necessarily one of the complementary therapies. It should be readily appreciated, therefore, that it is both intended and taken as read that proper supportive measures and other orthodox techniques of therapy should be used in serious diseases or syndromes, such as collapse, meningococcal meningitis, gross haemorrhage and severe schizophrenia. To the treatment of such major or life-threatening conditions the Formulary is only a complement, albeit a valuable one. I have also assumed that any effective orthodox medication will not be stopped abruptly without proper advice being taken, and that, in all problematical or serious cases, appropriate referral to those with greater expertise will be made. Furthermore, in **The Formulary** proper, I occasionally use such expressions as 'adjunctive therapy of', just to remind the reader that there are other things to be considered which are not covered by this book, be they commonly known (such as the low cholesterol diet) or of a decidedly professional orthodox nature (such as the use of insulin in diabetes).

Apart from these words of caution, and to emulate the words of the great Schnozzle Durante, this is not the book with which 'to prop up the short leg of your pool table'; nor, indeed, to grace the coffee table - as so many of a more domestic or academic inclination might seem to many of us 'in the business'.

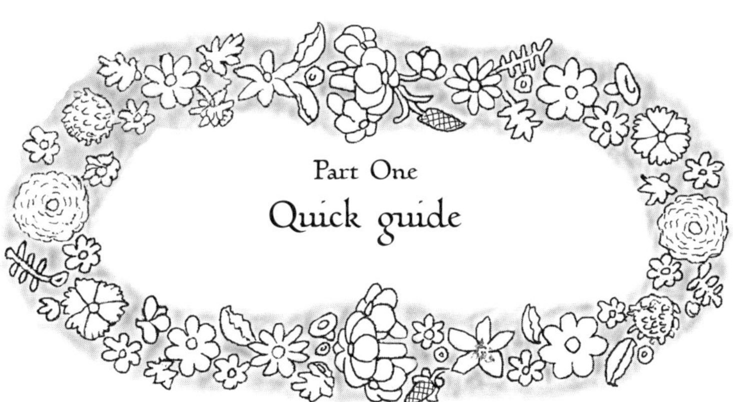

Part One

Quick guide

A quick guide to the use of the formulary

This **Complementary Formulary** should enable you to select prescriptions with some rapidity in busy pharmaceutical or clinical situations.

The rubrics refer to either diseases or syndromes, alphabetically listed and with adequate cross-reference.

Against each rubric is listed a limited number of specially selected **therapeutic entries**, sometimes followed by a brief extra **note**.

These listed **entries** are denoted by particular **icons**, for speedy identification of the type of therapy suggested and any additional notes:

- **Nutritional supplements** [Icon: the reclining chilli].
  Unless otherwise stated, the doses quoted are those for an adult. In the case of children, dosage of internally administered substances must be modified according to weight. As a general rule, where several such supplements are listed, they may be given either singly or in combination. They may also be usefully combined, if so desired, with any other suggested therapeutic agents. Although they have a high level of safety, Appendix 2 should be checked for any possible adverse interactions with other therapeutic substances (drugs or herbs) or contraindications, as appropriate. Large doses should not be given in pregnancy. Most nutritional substances are taken after food, but there are several important exceptions (e.g. amino-acids, Florisene®, NADH, Moducare®, chitosan). However, in these cases, the manufacturer's instructions will usually clarify the matter.

❀ **Herbal (Botanic) preparations** [Icon: the flower].
Unless otherwise stated, the doses quoted are those for an adult. In the case of children, dosage of internally administered substances must be modified according to weight. In the case of liquid preparations, the symbol Ø means mother tincture. The numerical expression that precedes it (e.g. 1:5) refers to the way it was prepared, expressing the weight/volume ratio of the herb/tincture in g/ml. The quoted dose for a 1:5 Ø must thus be doubled if only a 1:10 Ø is available. FE refers to fluid extract, which is essentially a 1:1 Ø. Therefore, where only a 1:10 Ø is available, when the text states FE, the number of drops to be given is 10 times that stated. Conversely, where the text states 1:10 Ø, and only a FE is available, the dose will be one tenth of that quoted. Standardized extracts, in the form of capsules or tablets obviously get over this problem. Some are to be found in the text, but they are not obtainable for every botanic medicine mentioned. Nevertheless, provided material is obtained from a reputable source, you can feel free to substitute any herbal preparation quoted with an alternative form; although you may then be obliged to follow the manufacturer's or supplier's directions as to dosage.

Unless otherwise stated, a cautious initial approach is to give only one internal botanic medicine for any particular case. That, however, may be usefully combined with any other therapeutic measures suggested, even herbal topical agents. Although they have a high level of safety, Appendix 2 should be checked for any possible adverse interactions with other therapeutic substances (drugs or herbs) or contraindications, as appropriate. Their use in pregnancy or lactation is best restricted to those with proper experience, with the exception of a few listed in the text for the treatment of certain conditions arising in relation to these matters. It may be assumed that most internal herbal substances are best taken after/with food with/in a little water, unless stated otherwise in the text or by the supplier (see also Section 2 in Part Two).

⚔ **Homoeopathic remedies** [Icon: the crossed swords of the Meissen porcelain factory, where Hahnemann's father worked as an artist - here symbolizing 'like cures like'].
The dose for an adult is the same as that for a child. A standard dose is one pilule, tablet, drop (liquid potency), or small pinch of powder or fine granules. The weight or size of the patient is irrelevant. Hence, in the text, these aspects of dosage are always the same, and taken as read (bar a limited number of

indicated exceptions). Most of the remedies quoted are those prepared on the centesimal scale of serial dilution and energization - hence the suffix c (e.g. 6c=6th centesimal potency). A few, however, are those manufactured on the decimal scale - hence the prefix D (e.g. D6=6th decimal potency). From a practical point of view, however, it is permissible to use a D preparation in substitution for a c, and vice versa - hence, in essence, 6c≡D6. Although a remedy may be quoted in a particular potency (e.g. 30c), it may be that the one in stock is different. In that case, provided that the available potency is lower (but not <6c/D12 for a toxic substance), it is permissible initially to substitute one for the other, whilst maintaining the same suggested frequency of dose repetition. This may be done until the indicated potency is obtained, whereupon it may be replaced - but only if necessary, as indicated by poor response. Higher potencies than those stated may cause some unwarranted side-effects, and are best avoided by those of lesser experience. See also my note on possible problems with the use of Silicea under 'Foreign bodies'. As a general rule, unless otherwise stated (and in treating an acute on chronic disease), only one homoeopathic remedy should be given at a time. However, large brackets {:::} indicate that a combination or prepared mixture of remedies is suggested. Nevertheless, a selected homoeopathic prescription may be combined usefully with any other suggested therapeutic measure.

Adverse interactions with drugs, herbs or nutritional substances are extremely rare and usually of little consequence. However, where a remedy is effective, the requirement for orthodox medication may be reduced. Mostly, the stated remedies are safe in pregnancy and lactation; but those that require infrequent repetition - such as once or twice weekly, fortnightly or monthly - should not be given in pregnancy without taking professional advice. Homoeopathic remedies are most frequently given on the tongue and at least 10 minutes away from food. In view of its possible antidotal action, coffee in any form is generally disallowed. Homoeopathic remedies can sometimes be prescribed merely on their correspondence to the average disease or syndrome pattern. Other times, a consideration of the broad characteristics of the patient (e.g. personality, reaction to temperature) or the particular symptoms and signs arising in the course of the disease must be taken into consideration for a prescription to be successful. In cases such as this, the information given after the remedy in small brackets {...} must be carefully considered, such as: '{shy}', '{hot}', '{with discharge}'. Note, however, that the qualification '{in general}' indicates that the highest priority should be given to that particular prescription.

Bach Flower Remedies [Icon: the radiant flower].
These have similarities to homoeopathic remedies in certain respects. They are usually given in liquid form, but do not bear a numerical indication of potency. The standard dose is 4 drops, irrespective of age, size or weight; and is generally taken as read throughout the text. Adverse interactions with drugs are extremely rare. They are prescribed upon the basis of psychological syndromes (e.g. 'Family, over-concern with'), and may be mixed together to cover a complex case; although, for those new to the subject, I do not recommend exceeding 3 in all. Where more than one is quoted, then each is followed by a brief note in small brackets {...} to aid selection, e.g. '{fears failure}'. They may also be given freely alongside homoeopathic remedies, and any other suggested therapeutic measure. They are extremely safe in both pregnancy and lactation. They are generally given on the tongue and preferably at least 10 minutes away from food.

Nutritional or Homoeopathic injections [Icon: the invasive dagger].
In this text, there are only two types listed: Vitamin B12 and sterilized injectable homoeopathic remedies. Both are extremely safe, incurring no interactive problems with other therapeutic agents. Nevertheless, Vitamin B12 injections can cause headaches in some people, and must then be abandoned. They are not to be recommended in pregnancy. Also the dose of B12 for children must be calculated from the stated adult dose according to weight. Where Vitamin B12 injections are recommended, they may always be usefully combined with any oral therapy. Thus, in treating, say, Bell's palsy (q.v.) or glandular fever (q.v.), it is important to give something medicinal by mouth at the earliest possible opportunity, even though injections of Vitamin B12 are being given concurrently. Where homoeopathic injections are recommended, it may be assumed that their action may be fortified by the concurrent administration of oral homoeopathic remedies, or, indeed, any other therapeutic agent. Furthermore, the stated volume to be administered is not usually critical, and may be reduced to one half in small persons or those with little subcutaneous fat.

ⓘ **General information** [Icon: i for information].
Some extra points of interest or relevance. Words that are underlined lead you to other relevant rubrics.

The list of therapies entered against each rubric is to be viewed rather like the menu in a restaurant. What is served depends on the availability of the food and the requirements (and sometimes the financial resources) of the client. Now, it would be most unusual for a single person to order everything on an extensive menu for himself. That would be gluttony. So, neither should we automatically prescribe everything listed in one go. Furthermore, most people would not order two or three soups. Most would prefer one. Similarly, we should be wary, at least initially, about giving two or more different oral homoeopathic prescriptions concurrently or, indeed, two or more internal botanics. Now, if we are in a real hurry or quandary, the best thing is to order the item on the top of the menu, where it has been deliberately placed as something of high therapeutic priority - unless there is information in small brackets that suggests otherwise in the case at hand. With regard to lists of Bach Flower Remedies, the consideration of any information in small brackets is always essential for correct selection.

Nevertheless, there are many rubrics, where the number of entries is sufficiently limited to make selection a good deal more simple.

In treating chronic diseases, it is wise to try out any item or items for at least one month before modifying the prescription. In acute disease, however, the prescription may require alteration every 1–7 days, according to response. The treatment of an acute condition should usually be stopped 24–48 hours after the patient appears to be totally free of symptoms (or upon recovery in ultra-acute disorders, e.g. collapse, acute epistaxis).

Where an acute illness occurs during a course of treatment for chronic disease, it is generally unwise to stop the latter. The temporary addition of an acute treatment to a chronic seldom causes problems, even if it means prescribing more than one homoeopathic remedy or botanic at the same time (see Section 3 in Part Two, for some rare homoeopathic exceptions).

As experience is gained, however, it will become apparent that the deliberate and cautious mixing of several homoeopathics or several botanics can produce some rather fine results in the treatment of both acute and chronic disease (hence, the suggested mixtures in some parts of the text). For the moment, those who lack proficiency should stick to the rules given.

Complementary medicine, rather like a game of chess, has many ways of winning.

An example from the text to illustrate practical prescribing

Acne vulgaris

- ❀ Smilax spp. 1:5 Ø 30gtt bd/tds.
- ❀ Vitex agnus-castus standardized 10:1 extract 100mg om.
- ⨯ Kali bromatum 6c bd {in general}.
- ⨯ Selenium 6c bd {with many comedones}.
- ⨯ Antimonium tartaricum 6c bd {with much pitting and scarring}.
- ➶ Zinc 15mg om/bd.
- ⓘ Where long-term antibiotics have been used, treatment for chronic gastrointestinal candidiasis may also be required.

This implies that Smilax, as top of the list, should be a good first choice - but let's assume that we cannot get any for quite a few weeks. So, we decide to consider the herbal alternative Vitex (although, equally, we might have decided to begin with one of the homoeopathic alternatives). This we obtain and give for one month. There seems to be some improvement, but we wish to fortify its action. Looking down the list, we see that three homoeopathic remedies appear in sequence. Kali bromatum is qualified by '{in general}', so we choose that. Unfortunately, things are not progressing too well with this combination after a further month. We decide to keep Vitex going, but prescribe Antimonium tartaricum, since there is 'much pitting and scarring'. Things are finally moving after yet another month, albeit slowly. We add some zinc, and look into the matter of possible chronic candidiasis. In the meantime, the Smilax Ø has finally arrived, but we hold it in reserve.

Abbreviations used in the text with examples

Abbreviated form	*Unabbreviated form*
6c	6th centesimal potency
D6	6th decimal potency
M	1000th centesimal potency
1gt	1 drop
10gtt	10 drops
2 cap	2 capsules
2 tab	2 tablets
30ml	30 millilitres
1000µg	1000 micrograms
20mg	20 milligrams
50g	50 grams
6kg	6 kilograms
250IU	250 international units
ung	Ointment
Ø	Mother tincture
FE	Fluid extract
2h	To be given every 2 hours
10m	To be given every 10 minutes
prn	When required
om	To be given every morning
on	To be given every night
bd	To be given twice daily
tds	To be given thrice daily
qds	To be given four times daily
inj	Injection
sc	To be given subcutaneously
im	To be given intramuscularly
/	or

Anglo–American spelling

There are quite a few variations in transatlantic spelling. This formulary has been arranged alphabetically largely in accordance with UK usage. Thus, North American readers may find the following table helpful:

USA/Canada	*UK*
Amebiasis	Amoebiasis
Anemia	Anaemia
Anesthesia	Anaesthesia
Apnea	Apnoea
Celiac	Coeliac
Diarrhea	Diarrhoea
Dysmennorrhea	Dysmenorrhoea
Edema	Oedema
Esophagitis	Oesophagitis
Galactorrhea	Galactorrhoea
Hemangioma	Haemangioma
Hematoma	Haematoma
Hemorrhage	Haemorrhage
Hemorrhoids	Haemorrhoids
Homeopathy	Homoeopathy
Hypercholesterolemia	Hypercholesterolaemia
Hypertriglyceridemia	Hypertriglyceridaemia
Hypoglycemia	Hypoglycaemia
Lymphedema	Lymphoedema
Myxedema	Myxoedema
Seborrheic	Seborrhoeic
Skepticism	Scepticism
Sulfate	Sulphate
Sulfoxide	Sulphoxide
Sulfur	Sulphur

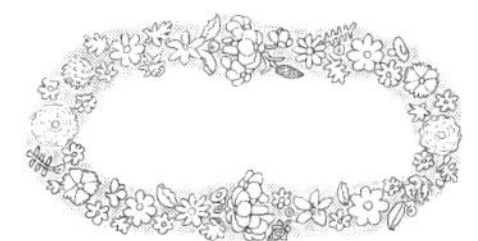

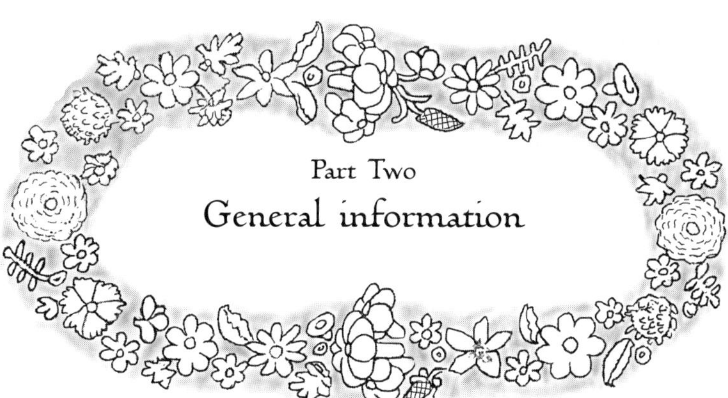

Part Two
General information

Section 1

Nutritional supplements

Nutritional therapy may involve either subtracting components from the diet or adding them. Removing or reducing nutrients is an important aspect of modern medical practice. You will all be familiar with many basic dietetic principles used in connection with various common conditions, such as diabetes mellitus and hypercholesterolaemia. For this reason, such discussions are not to be found in the text. However, you may be less familiar with those dietetic concepts useful in the treatment of, say, chronic candidiasis, chronic catarrh, reactive hypoglycaemia or inflammatory arthritis. Such things are included at the end of any appropriate entry in **The Formulary** proper. They may be taken as either simple information or indications for action, according to your own wishes and your professional situation with regard to the individual so afflicted. Nevertheless, any sensible exclusions should always allow for the possible consequential development of deficiency states, which must be opposed, either by dietetic rebalancing or nutritional supplementation.

In fact, supplements are of great benefit in an enormous number of conditions. Nutrients may be deficient because of inadequate diet, poor absorption, increased demands in the course of a disease (acute or chronic), failure of the local blood supply to deliver them, or impairment of the cellular wall transfer mechanisms. Indeed, one part of the body may have plenty, another, not enough. Thus, deficiencies can either be general or local. The hypertrophic prostate may be low in zinc, whilst the blood is replete with it. Iron deficiency, common in younger women with diffuse alopecia, often coexists with a normal blood-film. Furthermore, unless these deficiencies are corrected, nothing tends to get better. Deficiencies may be either acute, as with zinc and Vitamin C during a cold or fasting, or chronic, as with Vitamin E in varicose veins.

A *nutrient* may be roughly defined as a substance absorbed via the gut, other than water, which is utilized in the growth or maintenance of the *healthy* organism (drugs are thus excluded). Nutritional supplementation comprises giving larger quantities of nutrients than are normally found in the diet, or, by extension, those things which influence their absorption, either positively (e.g. digestive enzymes) or negatively (e.g. chitosan). Most supplements mix well with others, and with orthodox medication, herbal medicines, homoeopathy and Bach Flower Remedies. There are, however, a few problems which might be encountered, and these are indicated in Appendix 2 of Part Four. They include: the ill-effects of oily supplements in gallbladder disease; the production of subacute combined degeneration of the spinal cord where Vitamin B12, rather than Folic Acid, should have been given; the antidotal action of Folic Acid upon Phenytoin; and the affect upon congestive heart failure of abruptly withdrawing Coenzyme Q10.

There are two main sins in the provision of supplements - over-prescription and under-prescription. With regard to the former, there are some supplements, such as Vitamins A and D, which are positively toxic when given in large quantities. Most of us know the notorious Polar Bear liver story. Toxicity aside, there is also the ethical issue of unnecessarily emptying the wallet of the purchaser. Under-prescription, on the other hand, is safe, but equally stupid. This generally arises from either a lack of comprehension of effective dosage, or, in the case of expensive substances, from a wish to conserve finance. Many women who think they need relatively cheap Evening Primrose Oil take 500mg daily, which is but a drop in the proverbial ocean. Others with osteoarthritis take a mere 500mg daily of the relatively expensive supplement Glucosamine sulphate, despite perhaps being told that 1g is the minimum requirement for efficacy. Nevertheless, there is a certain leeway in prescribing, provided that dosages do not veer too sharply from those given in the text. Most supplements are perfectly satisfactorily given by mouth, but, with regard to therapeutic Vitamin B12, it is often better given by injection. Where injection is suggested in the text, it means *injection*, and implies that oral administration is a waste of time. Obviously, this puts the prescription out of the hands of the pharmacist. Quite apart from the treatment of pernicious anaemia, injectable Vitamin B12 has many, profound and varied clinical uses, as you will see upon consulting **The Formulary** proper in Part Three of this book. Although it occasionally causes headaches and must thus be stopped, above all, it is eminently safe, even in very high dosages. However, neither injections of Vitamin B12, nor large dosages of any oral nutritional substance are to be recommended in pregnancy.

Most supplements are best given after/with food, but there are a few notable exceptions, usually made clear by the supplier's literature. These include: various amino-acids, Florisene®, Moducare®, chitosan and NADH. The dosages given in **The Formulary** proper, unless otherwise indicated, are for adults, and must be reduced for children according to weight. A good general rule is to give one fifth of the stated adult dose for each 10kg (22lb).

Occasionally, you will encounter difficulties with vegetarians, vegans, various religious groups or BSE-paranoids who express concerns about gelatine capsules. You may find they accept removing the contents as an alternative, or you must find them tablets, powders or preparations encapsulated with vegetable materials. The latter, regrettably, are generally more expensive. The more adventurous of you might like to consider going back to pill-rolling.

Further reading

Werbach, M. R. *Nutritional Influences on Illness*. Third Line Press, 1993.

Murray M. T. and Pizzorno, J. E. *An Encyclopaedia of Natural Medicine*. Macdonald Optima, 1990.

Section 2
Herbal medicines

Herbal or botanic medicine is as old as the hills. Indeed, it can be regarded as the archetype of both current orthodox medicine and homoeopathy. Whilst herbalism utilizes material dosages of the whole of the appropriate part of the plant, and homoeopathy uses the same but infinitesimally, orthodox medicine, on the other hand, attempts to extract the principle; yet, like herbalism, applies it in significant measures. Practically, therefore, herbalism, although lying somewhere between the two other disciplines, is probably better regarded as a crude, yet useful, form of orthodoxy, incurring the same potential problems with toxicity.

Despite this general appraisal, many herbal medicines are remarkably safe, and are often effective where the orthodox will fail. Otherwise we would have no use for them, and most would have disappeared into a pharmaceutical grave long since. Those incorporated in **The Formulary** proper have been selected for their relative safety and efficacy. However, you should consult Appendix 2 of Part Four in order to determine any possible adverse interactions, side-effects or contraindications for those administered internally. Many mix quite well with orthodox drugs, homoeopathy, Bach Flower Remedies, nutritional supplements and other botanics (although I do not recommend that those new to the subject indulge in too much herbal polypharmacy). Since the *topically* applied herbs suggested in **The Formulary** proper generally incur only local adverse reactions (and then, only rarely), and seldom induce any problems from their minimal systemic absorption, they are deliberately *excluded* from Appendix 2; this matter being taken as read. Chinese herbs are mainly omitted in the current text, except for Ginseng, or where the plant is also part of western herbalism.

Most herbal preparations are best taken after food, both to slow their absorption and prevent gastric irritation; bar, especially, Vitex, which should be given upon rising, Ginger (Zingiber) for its antidyspeptic and antiemetic qualities, and Ulmus fulvus for ulcerative colitis. The doses quoted, unless stated otherwise, are for adults, and must be reduced for children according to body weight. The rule given in Section 1 for the dosage of supplements applies equally here.

Herbal medicines may be purchased in a variety of forms. These include: dried plant material, tablets, capsules, tinctures and fluid extracts. Each of these is represented in **The Formulary** proper, but the pharmacist or practitioner must feel free to switch between what I have suggested and any other reliably sourced preparation that is either more readily available or better suited to his style or that of the person to be treated. In that case, the directives concerning dosage (and any preparation) will usually be provided by the supplier; although this is also available via the websites given at the end of Appendix 2, or professional databases.

This brings us, quite appropriately, to the matter of standardization in herbal pharmacy, since dosage means very little unless we first qualify our products with statements concerning strength. What is five drops of one batch of nettle extracted in alcohol, might be equivalent to ten of another. With this problem in mind, I have deliberately prefixed each *mother tincture sign* Ø with a numerical expression, e.g. 1:5; in this case meaning that every 5ml of the original unfiltered tincture contained 1g of plant material. Roughly speaking, we may say that a 1:10 Ø is half as strong, and warrants a doubling of dosage as suggested for the 1:5. Yet, even this only goes part of the way towards standardization, since the chemical quality of the original plant material is subject to some variation according to location, soil, climate, water content and so on. Nevertheless, provided that the herbal tincture is obtained from a reliable source, its properties will generally remain clinically consistent; and, despite the theoretical objections, the dosage (and any indicated adjustment) will usually apply to a reasonable degree to any so procured, irrespective of manufacturer. Beyond that, there has always been some criticism levelled against *the drop* as a unit of measurement. Obviously, the size of the drop will vary slightly according to the dropper itself. In actual practice, however, neither this factor, nor those discussed previously, seem to make a significant difference to the clinical outcome in many situations. In fact, provided the tincture is of low toxicity, there will usually be more room for variation of absolute chemical dosage than holds with orthodox medication. In any case, it is usually simple enough to adjust the suggested dosage by small increments (1–3 drops) according to response. A *fluid extract* (FE), by the way, is essentially equivalent to a 1:1 Ø. Both tinctures and fluid extracts are usually taken in a little water after food and are generally relatively inexpensive.

We could, of course, as favoured by the Chinese, prepare decoctions of fixed weights of dried herbs by boiling. Rather like tinctures and fluid extracts, they are more readily and thoroughly absorbed than tablets and capsules. However, their preparation is often tiresome and the results excessively unpalatable. Nevertheless, there are certain additional, though minor, qualities acquired by boiling, which are essentially homoeopathic in nature; and more shall be said of this when we come to consider the Bach Flower Remedies in Section 4.

Compressed tablets or capsules containing known weights of the dried herb are another way of attempting to standardize. Despite the fact that drying removes the problem of assessing the water content of the original herb, it does nothing to solve that of variations in chemical composition. To this end, many botanic substances are now assayed for the content of what seems to be the main chemical principle, and some are even presented in an extracted form. Thus, we may have a tablet or capsule containing, say, a guaranteed 500 μg of hypericin. And, indeed, this is important with this particular substance, since it is hypericin that likely does all the work in Hypericum. However, such a methodology cannot be applied to all herbs, in that many of them work upon the basis of a synergism between several or many individual chemical components; a matter which still requires considerable elucidation. It should also be reiterated that dried or extracted forms are not necessarily so well absorbed as the liquid varieties, and some might feel that the latter are best; Feverfew being a notable exception, where the tincture, as opposed to the dry form, appears to be clinically inert in the treatment of migraine. That tinctures can occasionally be notably different from the raw plant is also illustrated by Poison Ivy (Rhus toxicodendron), where even the slightest contact with the fresh juice induces a vicious dermatitis via the chemical urushiol. In contrast, the alcoholic extract is devoid of urushiol activity, and may be incorporated in creams for the treatment of osteoarthritis.

Despite all these problems, herbs are of much use in clinical practice, and not as difficult to prescribe as might initially be thought. As far as their use in pregnancy and lactation is concerned, mostly they should be avoided by those who are other than expert. There are, however, a f exceptions to this rule given in the text. Ginger is particular teresting in this respect, in that it would seem to be an abor ient when given in large doses. However, in small doses it is only good to eat, but also particularly helpful in the treatment norning sickness. Upon this note, it is worth remarking that th s such as Ginger and Garlic are flavourings, foods and herbal edies all rolled into one, and thus cannot be exactly categoriz Quite arbitrarily, therefore, in **The Formulary** proper I have ssified Ginger as a herb and Garlic as a nutritional substance d would not argue with anyone who disagreed. Nevertheless, ough Garlic is not an essential nutrient to the English, it app that life in Mainland Europe and Korea cannot exist without

Some may be intrigued the strange sign Ø for *mother tincture*. In fact, it is the est standard typological equivalent (Greek Phi) to an ancient yric sigil, meaning 'spirit', 'essence' or 'essential principle'; an still in common use in homoeopathic pharmacy. Indeed, the al form 'spirits' for strong alcohol is derived from this notio is also interesting to observe that the alcohol-water used to act the plant is traditionally known as the *menstruum*. To old chemists, the process of extraction was highly feminine orm of giving birth to the spirit of the plant. Further details ne preparation of tinctures are to be found in Section 3, which ows, plus other comments concerning the use of alcohol in a olism and those of certain religious convictions.

Further reading

Werbach, M. R. and ay, M. T. *Botanical Influences on Illness*. Third Line Press, 1994.

Newall, C. A., Anderson, L. A. and Phillipson, J. D. *Herbal Medicines*. Pharmaceutical Press, 1996.

Section 3
Hom(o)eopathic remedies

To some, homoeopathy is a subject of mystery, to be regarded with great suspicion. This, however, is not due to any lack of clinical or experimental corroboration of its efficacy, but often rather to an inability to comprehend its physical basis. Hopefully, Appendix 3 of Part Four, concerning the detailed Physics of Homoeopathy will go some way towards rectifying this matter. However, it is best left in abeyance for the moment, whilst we consider some more basic pharmaceutical, clinical and historical concepts.

What is homoeopathy?

Homoeopathy may be defined as that school of medicine founded by Dr. [Christian Friedrich] Samuel Hahnemann, the medicinal therapeusis of which differs markedly from that of orthodox medicine, or *allopathy*, as he so termed it.

Who was Hahnemann?

Samuel Hahnemann was born at Meissen in Germany in 1755, where his father was a talented artist at the famous porcelain factory. Hahnemann was a chemist, physician, polyglottal translator and medical reformer. Appalled by the illogical, and often harmful, orthodox practices of the day, he sought to discover better and safer ways of prescribing medicines. His first major work on homoeopathic ideology, the *Organon der rationellen Heilkunde*, was published at Dresden in 1810. The 6th and final edition of this book, however, although completed a year or so before his death in Paris in 1843, remained generally unknown until 1921 (although an 'unofficial' version was apparently produced and circulated in limited edition by Dr. Arthur Lutze in 1865).

What is Hahnemann's fundamental proposition?

Hahnemann's fundamental proposition, now peculiar to homoeopathy, may be expressed thus:

> That the selection of a drug to treat a particular disease in the sick individual should be determined by its ability to induce a *similar* disease in the healthy.

This proposition is termed the *Law of Similars*, more concisely expressed in Latin as '*Similia similibus curentur*' ('Let likes be treated with likes'). The implication of this 'law' is that lesser doses have the opposite effect of greater.

Whereas other authors, including the illustrious Hippocrates himself, had suggested the occasional use of drugs upon an analogous basis, it was for Hahnemann to transform this proposition into the foundation for an extensive and valuable therapeutic system, which we term *homoeopathy**.

Toxicity and the Law of Similars

An important aspect of the Law of Similars, which has been established empirically, is that it continues to hold true even as the material therapeutic dose is considerably reduced. This matter is highly significant with regard to essentially toxic materials, such as *mercury*, where sub-toxic doses may still exert a curative effect.

*The derivation is from the Greek: ΟΜΟΙΟΣ, homoios, 'resembling'; and ΠΑΘΟΣ, pathos, 'that which happens (to a person)'. Hence, *homoeopathy* is 'the system of treating with something which has been shown to produce a state *resembling* that which happens'. In contrast, ΑΛΛΟΣ, allos, 'other', implies 'lacking similarity' (Latin: *alius*). Thus, *allopathy* (conventional medicine) is 'the system of treating with something which is incapable of generating a state similar to that which happens'. The word ΠΑΘΟΣ embraces not only 'disease' but also 'disorder', and thus includes such subtleties as changes in mood and sense of well-being.

An example of the application of the Law of Similars

The symptoms of *mercury* poisoning include halitosis, gingivitis and periodontitis. In accordance with the Law of Similars, homoeopathically prepared *Mercurius solubilis*, given in non-toxic quantities, may be used to treat some (but not all) types of gingival or periodontal disease. I shall say more of homoeopathic pharmaceutical technique later, but, for the moment, please note that the homoeopathic version of the drug, with few exceptions, is generally in a *latinized* form, in accordance with established international custom.

More about cause and cure

The picture of *disease* induced by the action of a drug is termed its *pathogenesis*. It includes both psychological and physical objective and subjective symptoms, and pathological and physiological changes. The pathogenesis is established by recording the effects generated by the drug when it is administered either accidentally or intentionally. An important type of intentional administration is the so-called homoeopathic *experimental proving*, where a drug is administered to a number of *healthy* human volunteers, who subsequently document the changes experienced; for which purpose, the drug is administered either in a crude form or as an attenuated homoeopathic preparation ('sporadic/clinical proving' may also occur during actual treatment, when the patient generates new and unusual symptoms related to the medicine given). The results of *provings* (experimental and sporadic), together with the symptomatic and pathological details recorded in cases of accidental or malicious poisoning (viz. *toxicology*), constitute the basis of the homoeopathic *materia medica*. When you read about symptoms or diseases in works of homoeopathic material medica, you must realize that it is implied that the relevant drug may either *cause* or *cure* the listed abnormalities, according to circumstances and dosage. Further on, I shall examine the structure of the material medica, and discuss how it has been (and *is being*) modified in the light of *clinical experience*.

What is 'the simillimum'

The closer the similarity between the documented pathogenesis of the drug and the disease picture of a particular patient, the more likely will that drug effect a cure in that patient. Drugs which exhibit such a close correspondence are said to be *homoeopathic* to the disease. The drug which is felt to have the greatest symptomatic and pathological correspondence is termed the *simillimum* (Latin: 'the *most* similar'), a more expansive definition of which will be provided later in the text. For the moment, let it be emphasized that the selection of the simillimum rests not only upon the orthodox diagnostic entity (the name of the disease) but, in many instances, also upon the individualized objective and subjective symptomatology (signs and symptoms respectively, as they are otherwise termed). Such symptomatic pictures may vary considerably between cases of disease within the same diagnostic category (e.g. influenza), with each case requiring a different simillimum. In other situations (such as the common traumatic bruise or dental abscess), the symptomatic response is more uniform, and the choice of a possible simillimum more limited, and hence simpler.

When is a drug not a drug?

Shortly I shall be discussing homoeopathic pharmaceutical preparation, one objective of which is the attenuation of toxicity of potentially harmful drugs. By definition, a *drug* is any non-nutritional substance used for its therapeutic action, be it current or obsolete; a term which, therefore, might even include attenuated homoeopathic preparations. However, common parlance supports our brief that homoeopathic attenuations should be termed *remedies* rather than *drugs*, the implication being that they are less noxious and immensely safer. Some, however, prefer to call them *medicines*, again implying something more benign.

From which classes of substance are remedies derived?

As I observed previously in **Section 2**, herbalism is the archetype for both homoeopathy and allopathy. Indeed, the first Hahnemannian remedy was China officinalis (Peruvian bark/Quinine), documented in 1796 (Hufeland's Journal, Vol. II, Jena). Nevertheless, contrary to popular notion, which confuses homoeopathy with herbalism, homoeopathic remedies are not solely derived from the vegetable kingdom, as you will have already gathered from my previous remarks concerning mercury. Many are prepared from minerals, and some from animal products, such as snake venoms. Between the animal and the vegetable kingdoms, bacteria, viruses, rickettsiae, protozoa and microfungi (or the tissues and exudates containing them) are transformed into remedies of the greatest therapeutic importance, termed *nosodes*; a designation which also includes any remedy from a diseased but uninfected tissue, such as cataract, osteoarthritic bone or carcinoma (a remedy made from a non-diseased tissue, such as a thyroid gland, is called a *sarcode*). Indeed, with certain exceptions (some of which are given in Appendix 3 of Part Four), one might say that virtually any matter or energetic radiation of the Universe might become a remedy, were its pathogenesis and therapeusis fully established. Even orthodox drugs have been used to create remedies. Perhaps more remarkably, homoeopathic pharmaceutical techniques can also unmask the therapeutic potential of substances which would normally be inert when administered by mouth (such as flint, yielding *Silicea*); their pathogenesis only becoming apparent in an attenuated form.

What is the objective of the pharmaceutical technique?

The objective of a homoeopathic pharmaceutical technique is twofold:

1. The attenuation of chemical toxicity.
2. The preservation, enhancement or development of medicinal action.

What are the stages of the pharmaceutical technique?

There are three to be described:

1. Selection and initial preparation.
2. Liquid phase potentization.
3. Medication.

Selection and initial preparation

Since many homoeopathic remedies are derived from herbaceous plants, it is appropriate that with these the method should be exemplified. Pre-eminently, the plants should be identified as being of the correct species, healthy and vigorous. They should be gathered in full bloom, and before overt seed formation; preferably on a bright morning after a rainy night. Under such circumstances they will be in their prime, and their pharmacological content generally optimal. Having washed them, the appropriate parts of the plants are selected, and finely chopped or minced. Sometimes the whole plant is utilized. The disrupted material is then macerated in ethanol–water in a tightly-stoppered glass vessel in a cool dark place, and agitated daily for 8 days or so. The selected strength of the alcoholic menstruum is generally 60–80%, being largely dependent upon the juice content of the plant material. The higher the water content of the material (as assayed by desiccation), the greater the strength of alcohol required.

The contents of the vessel are then decanted, strained and filtered, to yield the functional mother tincture, usually denoted by Ø (see the end of Section 2), or occasionally by the abbreviations MT or TM. This is stored in amber glass bottles in a cool dark place until ready to be subjected to the next stage of homoeopathic preparation, termed *potentization*.

Mother tinctures can be made from any substance soluble in ethanol–water. These include all manner of plant materials, some minerals (such as phosphorus, for which absolute alcohol is used), and various animal products (such as snake venoms). The preparation of these is delineated in various versions of the *homoeopathic pharmacopoeia*. The trend these days is very much towards standardization of procedure, in order to produce international uniformity of quality. Most mother tinctures have a shelf-life of approximately 5 years, after which time they should be discarded and replaced.

Within the mother tincture, the function of alcohol is to extract, modify and preserve. The solute which it contains is termed the *original substance*, and how this is *potentized* is the subject of the next discussion. For the moment, the preparation of substances *insoluble* in ethanol–water will be left in abeyance.

Liquid phase potentization

This unique process, peculiar to homoeopathy, consists of *serial dilution* together with the *application of mechanical energy* at each stage. It cannot be over-emphasized that it is not merely a matter of simple dilution alone.

Serial dilution implies that each dilution is of equal magnitude and is made from the one which immediately precedes it.

One drop of Ø is added to a glass vial containing 99 drops of ethanol–water (about 3.6ml; strength 15–95%, according to the pharmacy). The vial is stoppered and then violently agitated. This violent mechanical energy is termed *succussion*, and is more effectively carried out if the vial is no more than three-quarters full. Mechanical succussion devices are available, but the process is very simply carried out manually (for convenience, the instructions that follow are for right-handed operators).

Succussion actually consists of two phases: shaking and jolting. The vial is grasped in the palm of the right hand, with the thumb held firmly over the stopper. The vial is shaken well, each shake terminating in a jerk, achieved by striking the closed right hand (which protects the glass) against the open palm of the left hand. This is repeated, according to the custom of the pharmacy, 10–20 times. Rapping the bottom of the vial cautiously on a leather-bound book may be substituted for the use of the left hand. This completes the preparation of the *1st centesimal potency* or *attenuation*, which is labelled *1c*. The term *centesimal* refers to the serial dilution *scale* of 1 in 100.

One drop of the 1st centesimal potency or attenuation is then added to 99 drops of ethanol–water in a new vial with a fresh stopper, and this is succussed in the same manner as described previously. This yields the *2nd centesimal potency/attenuation*, which is labelled *2c*. The dilution is now 1 in 10,000 (1 in 10^4).

The processes of serial dilution and succussion continue thereafter in an identical fashion; so by the time we have prepared the potency of 30c, we have 30 stoppered vials, labelled from 1c to 30c, the dilution of the latter being 1 in 10^{60}.

The process of potentization may be continued almost *ad infinitum*, although normally the highest potency produced is *CM* (=100,000c), corresponding to an extraordinary dilution of 1 in $10^{200,000}$.

With regard to remedies in general, the most frequently used potencies are 6c, 12c, 30c, 100c, 200c and M (=1000c). By convention, the suffix *c* is *often omitted*, so that, say, Arnica 30=Arnica 30c. In Mainland Europe you will also find the use of *cH* as an alternative to *c*. In **The Formulary** proper, to make things clear, the suffix *c* is always given. Very high potencies, such as 10M (=10,000c), 50M (=50,000c) and CM, are more conveniently prepared by a technique of potentization termed *Korsakov's method*, described below.

Later, I shall make mention of two other *scales* of dilution used in homoeopathy, the *decimal* and the *LM*.

Medication

The term *liquid potency* is applied to any homoeopathic attenuation in ethanol–water, irrespective of the scale of dilution. Such liquid potencies may be administered directly on the tongue in the form of drops, a technique particularly useful in the unconscious, semiconscious or very young. More commonly, however, various solid sugars (especially sucrose) are medicated with them (1 drop per 7–14g), these preparations being more convenient for general use. Remedies may thus appear in the form of powders, coarse and fine granules, spherical pilules and tablets.

What is Korsakov's method?

Essentially, this is serial potentization within a *single* glass vial. Instead of transferring one drop of the liquid potency to another vial of fresh diluent, the vial is emptied, leaving some of the liquid potency adherent to its inner surface. The conformation of the vial is such that approximately one drop remains. To the same vessel, 99 drops (about 3.6ml) of diluent are added, and succussion carried out in the normal way. Again the vial is emptied, more diluent added, and succussion applied. In this way, it is possible to carry out serial potentization without the need for large numbers of vials. In terms of alcohol, however, it is no more economical than the normal method.

The Korsakovian system is used in the case of automatic mechanical potentizers involved in the production of very high liquid potencies. In the Pinkus Potentizer, this is combined with the so-called Skinnerian method, where succussion and dilution are simultaneously produced by the force of the entering diluent; which, in this particular device, is effected by an intermittent forcible jet of ultra-pure water. There are 80 successive blows (against a Neoprene-rubber pad) per phase of serial dilution, this compounding with the energization produced by the Skinnerian hydraulic effect.

Potentization and medicinal action

One of the great controversies concerning homoeopathic remedies is the issue of their pharmacological effect in extreme dilution. At a dilution of 1 in 10^{12} (potency 6c), the molecular or ionic concentration of an original substance is so small that, in normal clinical dosage, even the most virulent poison is deemed to have negligible chemical toxicity. Futhermore, in dilutions in excess of 1 in 10^{24} (potency 12c), there are no traces of original substance whatsoever (except, perhaps, the odd molecule); hence the concept of the *infinitesimal dose*. However, both clinical and experimental evidence confirm that homoeopathic potencies in excess of 6c, and even 12c, do exhibit predictable pharmacological activity, and that their *placebo* effect is no greater than might be expected from any medicament, conventional or otherwise. In this respect, therefore, *succussed* potencies appear to be quite different from unsuccussed simple or serial dilutions.

The foundation for this peculiar phenomenon appears to be what is known as *water-memory*, and those who would like to learn more about its physics should consult Appendix 3 of Part Four.

What is the significance of 'potency'?

Although the dilution factor increases with the numerical value of potency, the therapeutic effects also increase, as a result of serial mechanical energization. The remedy becomes swifter in action and more eradicative of disease; in other words, stronger. At the same time, in many cases, its *range* is extended, so that profound physiological and biochemical effects may be experienced throughout the organism, including alterations in the psyche. Such may be termed a *constitutional response*, and the remedy given, a *constitutional remedy*. Not all remedies, however, routinely produce such widespread effects, even in high potency. Many, such as Ruta (for sprains), have a more restricted action on the physiology in virtually any potency, and may be described as *pathological remedies*. Lower potencies (e.g. 6c) of so-called constitutional remedies may also manifest such a restricted or pathological action (such as Pulsatilla for sties). The type of response (pathological or constitutional) is also dependent upon patient *sensitivity*; so that sensitive subjects may experience constitutional effects even with low potencies of either type of remedy. Nevertheless, with regard to general and common prescribing as delineated by **The Formulary** proper, whilst you should be made aware of this fact, it is a situation which will only occasionally arise.

For these reasons, it is better for those new to the subject not to exceed any potency given in **The Formulary** proper, should the stated one be unavailable. Lower ones, provided that they are not <6c or <D12 (see below) for toxic substances, are acceptable, and, for practical purposes, may initially be given with the same

suggested frequency of repetition. Remedies that are given *infrequently* (e.g. once or twice weekly, fortnightly) are of sufficient potency of action to be avoided by the less experienced in pregnancy (with the exception of Caulophyllum as a preparation for labour, prior to term).

What is the decimal scale?

This is serial potentization, where the dilution at each stage is 1 in 10, rather than 1 in 100. In order to distinguish them from centesimal scale preparations, decimal potencies are qualified either by the prefix D or the suffix x. Hence, D6=6x. In **The Formulary** proper, the D form is preferred, being clearer. The decimal scale is actually more popular in Central Europe; though, even in the UK and the USA, the *biochemic tissue salts* and lower potencies of insoluble substances (see below) are routinely prepared in this manner. In terms of therapeutic potency, the decimal scale may be regarded as slightly weaker than the centesimal. Thus, 30c has a more powerful action than D30. Yet, in practical terms, one could be substituted for the other.

Solid-phase potentization

Substances which are neither soluble in water nor ethanol (such as silica and mercury) are prepared by prolonged *trituration* (grinding) and serial dilution with lactose, using a ceramic mortar and pestle, or some equivalent mechanical device. The physics of this is also discussed in Appendix 3 of Part Four.

The *biochemic tissue salts* (not mentioned in **The Formulary** proper) are always prepared in this manner. By the time a potency in lactose of 3c or D6 (both of dilution 1 in 10^6) has been achieved, the original substance will have become colloidally suspensible in ethanol-water. Therefore, from 4c or D7 upwards, potentization proceeds in the *liquid phase*, as described previously. Below 4c or D7, the preparations are compressed into tablets. Since they are composed of milk-sugar, vegans will naturally object to them.

What is the LM scale?

This is rather a specialized scale in homoeopathy, and is not to be found in **The Formulary** proper. However, you should be made aware of its existence, since it has grown in popularity amongst homoeopathists. It was essentially unknown until 1921, when the 6th edition of Hahnemann's *Organon* became generally available.

Its fuller name is the *fifty millesimal scale*, since the degree of dilution at each stage is 1 in 50,000. The number of successions applied after each dilution is 100 (rather than 10–20). The scale is a little confusing, however, since LM1 is prepared in liquid phase as a 1 in 50,000 dilution from the 3rd centesimal *trituration* in lactose of either an insoluble or *soluble* substance. Mother tinctures as such are not required, the raw plant materials themselves sufficing; either in the form of the freshly squeezed sap preserved with alcohol, or as dried powders.

Again, you will find the physics of this process discussed briefly in Appendix 3 of Part Four. Even the low LM potencies are considerably more therapeutic than the numerically equivalent centesimal or decimal scale attenuations.

Are there other ways of preparing remedies?

Homoeopathic remedies may be *simulated* by various commercially available electromagnetic devices which implant 'patterns' upon ethanol-water. Not being the 'genuine article', they are, however, of little significance to the pharmacist. Their relationship to the norm is as that of the fake Rolex to the real McCoy. Both, of course, will tell the time. Nevertheless, their physics cannot be ignored, and is also covered in Appendix 3 of Part Four.

What constitutes a dose?

In general, except in the case of sensitive patients, a remedy may be considered to have a *trigger action*; that is to say, provided a certain minimum dose is given, dispensing a larger dose will not increase the effect. Generally, an increase in effect can only be produced by either giving a higher numerical potency or by repetition of the dose after a particular interval of time. In the oral administration of potentized remedies, which is by far the most common route, a single dose may be taken to be: *one* pilule, tablet, small pinch of fine granules, or drop of liquid potency (despite this, some manufacturers/prescribers recommend larger amounts, e.g. 2 pilules, 1 whole tube of fine granules; though this only fortifies the effect in the case of very sensitive subjects, and not routinely). This is the same for both adults and children, with the exception of compressed triturated lactose tablets (e.g. biochemic tissue salts, Sulphur D6/6x), where the dose is 4 tablets for an adult and 2 for a child. A drop of liquid potency or a small pinch of impregnated fine sugar granules are better suited to the treatment of children under 2 years of age, by avoiding the risk of pilule or tablet inhalation. Pilules and fine granules are composed of sucrose, whereas most tablets are composed of lactose. In cases of *lactase deficiency*, lactose-based preparations should be avoided. Lactase deficiency has an incidence of about 12.5% in northern and western Europeans, and of about 80% in American Indians, Asians, blacks and Mediterranean peoples. Sucrose intolerance is not unknown either, in which case neither pilules nor fine granules should be used. However, with regard to patients suffering from candidiasis, diabetes or reactive/non-diabetic hypoglycaemia, the quantity of sugar in a single dose is insufficient to cause any problems. However, the presence of even small doses of alcohol in pilules or tablets is sufficient to prohibit their use, and that of liquid alcohol potencies themselves, in the treatment of patients receiving *Antabuse* therapy for alcoholism. This may also cause problems with strict members of various faiths or followers of AA.

Rules for the administration and storage of remedies

These are very simple. Nevertheless, to save much time, trouble and your larynx, those relevant to the patient can be issued as a print-out:

1. All potentized remedies should be stored away from sunlight or artificial UV (as with mother tinctures), and perfumed substances or camphor in tightly stoppered vials (preferably made of amber glass). In glass, the shelf-life of correctly stored sugar-based remedies is probably no more than 5 years, and I would recommend discarding them after 2, and obtaining new stock. In plastic vials, the same preparations should be discarded after 1 year. Liquid potencies, however, stored correctly and in glass, have an almost indefinite shelf-life, provided that a single succussion is applied to them not less than once per month (or that they are kept in a drawer that is constantly opened and closed, or that they are in constant use for dispensing). Never let the remedies be stored in any cabinet that smells of oil of cloves or camphor, nor let them be exposed to any intense magnetic field. It is also a good idea to keep solid preparations away from intense sources of heat,

in that excessive dehydration may render them inert. Remedies are not affected by airport screening X-rays.

2. Solid remedies should not be directly handled, except momentarily. It is actually better that a pilule or whatever is jiggled from the vial into its lid or a clean teaspoon, and then given directly into the mouth. Special dispensers are sometimes available which deliver one pill at a time, and simplify the problem. Drops should be applied straight on the tongue with the dropper held at some distance. Solid remedies should be sucked, or crunched between the teeth and the fragments sucked. The action of the remedy may be delayed if such a remedy is immediately swallowed.
3. Neither food nor drink should be taken for 10 minutes before and after administration.
4. Peppermints and mint-flavoured toothpastes may interfere with the action of the remedy; but, provided that the 10-minute rule (as given above) is observed, they are unlikely to exert any significant negative effect.
5. Unconscious and semiconscious patients, and small children should only be given liquid potencies, *finely crushed* pilules (or tablets) or fine granules.
6. Dose repetition is determined by the nature and potency of the remedy, and the nature of the condition being treated. Severe acute conditions (e.g. collapse) generally require more frequent dose repetition.
7. *Coffee*, even when decaffeinated, may be strongly antidotal to the action of some remedies (especially Pulsatilla and Rhus toxicodendron) in some, but not all, persons, and according to the quantity consumed. It is thus best avoided generally during treatment. Ginger (Zingiber) seems to exert no inhibiting effect, provided that the 10 minute rule (given above) is observed, as with garlic, chilli or onions. Alcohol and tea in moderation are harmless.

Where and how do potentized remedies act?

This matter, almost as controversial as the physicochemical basis of potentization itself, is covered in Appendix 3 of Part Four.

Proving and aggravation during treatment

These terms are related. They apply to the situation where the remedy *produces* the subjective or objective symptoms which it normally *removes*. For example, a patient taking the remedy Natrum muriaticum for the prevention of cold sores may experience a gross increase in lesion pain, severe headache and intense thirst (such never having been experienced previously); all those symptoms being usually removed by the remedy. This often results from too high a potency being used (e.g. 200c), too frequent dose repetition (such as one dose every 2 hours), or extreme subject sensitivity. In such cases, the current remedy should be discontinued until things settle down, and the case reconsidered; later, either using the same remedy less aggressively (i.e. in lower potency or less frequently) or a new prescription altogether (or even nothing, if the cold sores do not recur). Technically, we should refer to an exaggeration of former symptoms (those related to the cold sore) as an *aggravation*, and the new symptoms developed by the remedy (headache and intense thirst) as a sporadic or clinical *proving*.

How are remedies selected?

As noted previously, remedies may have a generalized or *constitutional* effect, or a more restricted action on particular pathologies or biochemical dysfunctions. The latter is termed their *pathological action*, and, in this respect, the use of **The Formulary** proper is most appropriate.

The Formulary is what is termed a *therapeutic index*. This is an alphabetical index of diseases and syndromes classified in the orthodox or common manner; following which a number of different homoeopathic (and other) treatments is given under each diagnostic entity.

Although sometimes we are fortunate in having remedies which exhibit an exact correspondence with a particular orthodox category (e.g. Hepar sulph. in the subacute/chronic dental abscess), in many cases, in order to prescribe satisfactorily, the objective and subjective symptoms (signs and symptoms) individually manifest by the patient must be taken into consideration.

Although Chamomilla is almost routinely prescribed for infantile teething, it may fail in cases with excessive salivation, where Mercurius solubilis is better indicated. Even the character of a pain may be of some relevance: throbbing, stabbing, burning, crushing, and so on. The *laterality* of the symptoms may also determine the selection of the remedy; Sanguinaria being more commonly indicated in right-sided migraine and Spigelia in that involving the left side of the head. *Concomitant symptoms*, remote from the area of pathology, such as the occurrence of extreme restlessness with cold sores, may indicate one remedy rather than another (in this case, Rhus toxicodendron).

Also often warranting consideration are things or circumstances which make a complaint or a person better or worse (or feel that way). These are termed *modalities*. In this respect, homoeopaths have borrowed the symbols < and > from mathematics, meaning 'less than' and 'greater than' respectively. In homoeopathy, however, they are taken to mean 'worse/worse for' (<, lessening of health) and 'better/better for' (>, increase in health). Hence, 'toothache>cold water in mouth' means that cold rinses help the toothache. Modalities may be classified as:

1. Thermal: < or > heat or cold.
2. Climatic: e.g. < or > rain, storms, wind, snow, humidity, change in the weather.
3. Thermoclimatic: e.g. < humid heat, cold winds, hot rooms.
4. Periodic or Time: e.g. < after midnight, between 4 and 8pm, monthly, annually, in summer.
5. Kinetic or Positional: e.g. < or > movement, staying still, descent, lying on left side.
6. Nervous: e.g. < mental exertion, sunlight, strong odours, touch.

Remember that modalities can apply to the person in general as well as to any presenting complaint. Sometimes they appear paradoxical; for example, generally < cold, but headache > cold, suggests Arsenicum album.

N.B. In **The Formulary** proper, in order to avoid confusion, the symbols < and > are discarded in favour of normal English. However, since they are in such common use in homoeopathy, it is as well to understand what they mean.

Constitutional aspects of pathological prescribing

Experienced prescribers often utilize an assessment of the general or *constitutional* aspects of the patient to assist them in the prescription of an appropriate remedy. For example, Natrum muriaticum is better suited to a *hot* individual (feels generally < heat) than a chilly one (feels generally > heat). Sepia, however, is the opposite. Therefore, in the preventative treatment of cold sores, Natrum muriaticum will be better indicated for the hot woman, and Sepia for the chilly one. This is an example of the concept of *susceptible typology*; which essentially means that a certain type or person is sensitive to the action of a particular remedy or group of remedies.

Extending this concept, does this mean that Nat. mur. (as it is often so abbreviated) will have no effect upon the prevention of cold sores in a chilly person? This might be so; but, more likely, it will exert some effect, but less than it would in a hot type. The general constitution of the patient (which includes such parameters as thermal sensitivity, bodily conformation, colouring, pathological predispositions and personality) thus determines, in part, the efficacy of the pathological remedy. Hepar sulph., which almost routinely alleviates subacute or chronic dental abscesses in the majority, is actually most efficacious (swiftest in action) in those individuals who are flabby, chilly, hypersensitive to pain and easily angered. In other words, this is the *susceptible typology* for Hepar sulph., and the individual in whom it is manifest is said to be a 'Hepar sulph. type'. The constitution is named after a remedy to which it significantly corresponds. Similarly, we may talk of 'Phosphorus', 'Pulsatilla', 'Sulphur', 'Calcarea fluorica', 'Nat. mur.', and many other 'types'.

The 'pathological simillimum'

This is the remedy best indicated in terms of the individual symptomatology of the patient with regard to the presenting complaint; though sometimes with some partial consideration of the general or constitutional aspects of the case. It is *not*, in view of what has been said, the *only* remedy which will act on the pathology. There is, thus, a certain leeway in homoeopathic prescribing, where a remedy that is only partially indicated may still exert a certain beneficial effect. Hence, even when the most theoretically ideal remedy (the simillimum) is unavailable, a secondary remedy may often be selected, to great effect.

It should be emphasized that, whereas homoeopaths place great emphasis on individual symptomatology, the main action of the chosen pathological simillimum is upon the pathology itself. There is, however, some evidence (viz. its speed of action) that Arnica has some limited analgesic effect in cases of bruising or crushing.

Constitutional prescribing

This implies prescription based mainly upon the *general* aspects of the patient (see above), rather than those related to the presenting complaint; this beginning even as the patient enters for the first time, where such matters as general build, gait, colouring, tidiness, demeanour and cleanliness must be assessed. This aspect of prescribing is more relevant to the treatment of *chronic* disease, where it is, to some degree, functionally reversible by medicinal means (such as rheumatoid arthritis, eczema, predisposition to polypus formation). This usually requires much time spent with the patient, competent use of what is termed a *repertory* (see below), and is less suited to busy OTC (over-the-counter) or clinical situations. It often requires a large number of consultations or assessments (at monthly intervals or less) in order to achieve satisfactory results. Here, the *simillimum* with regard to the general or constitutional aspects of the patient, in some cases, may be difficult to assess with ease, and the 'cure' is often achieved by a sequence of 'simillima' over the course of many months.

Although it might seem somewhat illogical to relegate the presenting complaint of a person to a position of secondary importance, and to favour those aspects of the patient which *appear* to be unrelated to it, this is not the case. Viewing a particular disease as an unhealthy tree, and the basic physiology as the soil in which it grows, it follows that we may either spray the leaves of the tree directly (pathological prescribing), or treat it at the roots by modifying the soil (constitutional prescribing). Modifying the general physiology often produces more profound and lasting cures in chronic disease than is achievable with pathological prescribing alone. Ideally, a constitutional remedy should also cover the presenting complaint and its individualized symptoms. This, however, may be difficult to achieve with a single remedy. Hence, many chronic diseases are treated with some combination or alternation of both constitutional and pathological remedies.

Where a chronic disease is incurable, due to severe and irreversible anatomical change (e.g. gross osteoarthritis), or where the physiology is greatly weakened by malnutrition, chronic ill-health or age, it is often better to palliate the case with pathological remedies than to offer a constitutional prescription. In the case of severe anatomical change, little good will be achieved by a constitutional prescription. In the case of a weakened physiology, much strain will be placed upon it by such prescribing, which may, in itself, produce a further deterioration of the patient, with, in some cases, the necessity to supply an antidotal remedy (prescribed according to the symptomatology of the deteriorated state). This deterioration is caused by the deployment of energy to the treatment of a disease from an already depleted energy pool.

What is a repertory?

A *repertory* is quite different from a therapeutic index, such as **The Formulary** proper. Although it may have a limited number of entries concerning conventional diagnostic categories, these do not comprise its main substance; nor is its purpose to act as a mere substitute. The bulk of the repertory is concerned with individual objective and subjective symptoms (such as rash, pain in the face), qualifications of those symptoms (including character, modalities, laterality) and general aspects of the patient (such as thermal sensitivities, desires, aversions, food likes and dislikes, pathological predispositions, bodily conformation, colouring, emotional status, and so on). These are classified under various headings and subheadings, termed *rubrics*. Under each rubric a number of remedies is listed, using a variety of type faces (bold, italic, etc.) to denote grades of importance. The idea is to select a remedy that appears to be dominantly expressed throughout a large proportion of the selected rubrics. In fact, special numerical scoring methods are taught for this purpose. One of the better ones is Robin Murphy's *Homeopathic Medical Repertory*, which has a very satisfactory alphabetical arrangement. Nevertheless, those who wish to subjugate themselves to the gods Rom and Ram, will find that there are now a number of computer software packages available which help to accelerate the process of what is termed *repertorization*, i.e. the selection of a remedy via a repertory. However, repertorization is not suited to busy OTC or clinical situations (except in the case of those more expert), and the use of **The Formulary** proper, under these circumstances, is more appropriate.

The materia medica

There are numerous works on *materia medica*, where the remedies are listed alphabetically and their properties delineated under various headings: pathological indications, susceptible typology, mind, head, eyes, nose, face, mouth, stomach, abdomen, stool, urine, male, female, respiratory, heart, back, extremities, sleep, fever, skin, modalities, relationship and comparison with other remedies, and dosage. The one to be recommended to the busy pharmacist or professional prescriber as a good basic reference work is William Boericke's *Pocket Manual of Homoeopathic Materia Medica*.

Treated as a whole, the homoeopathic materia medica has many objective and subjective signs (pathogeneses), the clinical significance of which has never, or seldom, been verified. These are symptoms or signs which have been caused by a drug or potentized remedy (by proving or toxicity), but, although the implication is that they might also be cured by the relevant remedy, this has not been satisfactorily confirmed. Good works of materia medica, however, emphasize which diseases and syndromes have been repeatedly cured by a particular remedy, so that we may be more certain in our choice. Indeed, there are some entries where only the curative aspect of a remedy has been observed, and not the pathogenetic.

In homoeopathic prescribing, particularly at the constitutional level, much emphasis is often placed on the so-called *mentals*; so much so, that the *mentals* are separated from the *generals*. The term *mentals* refers to the detailed psychological status of the individual (such as weepiness, friendliness, etc.), which is often taken as a prime indication for the 'constitutional simillimum' (when an acute anxiety state in relation to, say, a dental procedure is treated as an entity in itself, this is a form of pathological, rather than constitutional prescribing).

Many of us feel, however, that the ideal selected constitutional remedy should not only cover the mental and general aspects of the case, but also those of the presenting complaint or pathology (and, preferably, with regard also to its individual symptomatic manifestation). Therefore, where two remedies would seem to be in contest on the basis of the mental and general analysis, that which more frequently treats the particular pathology should be selected in preference. In contrast to the generals, details concerning a particular pathology or disease (the presenting complaint), and its individualized objective and subjective symptoms, are termed the *particulars*.

What are leading symptoms?

A *leading symptom* is one that leads to the consideration of a limited number of remedies above all others; although often one of these is more commonly indicated, e.g. *excessive salivation and halitosis* with toothache→Merc. sol. (Mercurius solubilis). A leading symptom may, in fact, be a quality or modality, e.g. *throbbing* pain→Belladonna; toothache > *cold water in the mouth*→Chamomilla or Coffea cruda. These are leading symptoms in pathological prescribing, but the concept may also be applied to constitutional remedy selection, e.g. irritability < *especially to her nearest and dearest*→Sepia. Leading symptoms are also called *keynotes*.

However, when all is said and done, a remedy might be indicated for consideration by a leading symptom, but can only be selected as appropriate if it matches in other respects. Irritability towards one's husband, in itself, is not a sufficient basis for the prescription of Sepia; but, where it occurs in an overworked female with bearing-down feelings in the lower abdomen (sometimes from uterine prolapse), then it becomes strongly indicated. Some talk of a 'three-legged stool', implying that much good prescribing can be achieved by finding three *leading symptoms* which match a particular remedy. Indeed, in the hands of the expert prescriber, it is a valid and valuable technique. For those interested in pursuing this approach, E. B. Nash's *Leaders in Homoeopathic Therapeutics* is to be recommended for further reading.

Strange, *rare* or *peculiar* symptoms are a particular subgroup of leading symptoms, which have an enigmatic and inscrutable nature, and which lead to the consideration of particular remedies, e.g. burning sensation < *heat*→Arsenicum album; urgency to urinate < *putting hands in cold water*→Kreasotum.

Prescription by causation

Sometimes a remedy can be prescribed on the basis of the event, circumstances or disease which seemed to precipitate the presenting complaint or constitutional upset, even though this may have occurred many years previously. Frequently, the same remedy may be given as might have been possibly chosen for the precipitating disturbance itself. For example: epilepsy following concussion→Natrum sulphuricum (a principal remedy for concussion; not well since *mechanical trauma*→Arnica (a key remedy for mechanical trauma); not well since *BCG immunization*→BCG nosode; inflammatory arthritis from *dental focal sepsis*→Hepar sulph. (the principal remedy for chronic dental abscess).

What is isopathy?

This is simply the treatment of a disease with a remedy made from its presumed causative agent, e.g. Mixed regional pollens 30c for hay fever; House dust mite 6c for allergic rhinitis/sinusitis; Mercurius sol 6c for mercury toxicity; Meningococcinum 6c for meningococcal meningitis (to oppose the toxin). Other than their bearing on the matter of optimal potency, individual symptoms play no part in their selection (generally, the worse the symptoms, the higher the potency required, except in cases of toxicity, where lower potencies are preferable).

What is a polychrest?

This is a remedy of wide therapeutic applications, such as Pulsatilla, Arsenicum album, Phosphorus and Sulphur. Such remedies are important in the correction of the constitution in general, and also manifest important corrective effects on a wide variety of pathologies.

What is a miasm?

The term *miasm* (plural: miasm*s*/miasm*ata*) is applied to various diagnostic entities in homoeopathy:

1. A familial genetic trait (such as thyroid disease).
2. An inherited Lamarckian disease trait stemming from ancestral infection (e.g the tuberculous miasm from ancestral TB, which may lead to bronchitic tendencies in the descendants).
3. The prolonged aftermath of an infection or immunization (e.g. postviral syndrome, epilepsy following measles immunization, a tuberculous miasm following TB in the individual himself).
4. The prolonged aftermath of drug or chemical toxicity when the causative agent is no longer present in the body.

Remedies such as Bacillinum and Medorrhinum are essentially anti-miasmatic, and are generally given infrequently for the treatment of *chronic* disease. However, as you will note from **The Formulary** proper, Medorrhinum is also an *acute* remedy in its own right for the treatment of acute otitis media and the prevention of barotrauma.

What is Hering's Law?

Constantine Hering was one of Hahnemann's more important pupils. *Hering's Law*, which first appeared in a preface to Hempel's translation of Hahnemann's *Chronic Diseases* (Vol. I) in 1845, gives us the means of assessing the correct progression of curative (constitutional) treatment of a *chronic* disease:

Cure occurs from above downwards, from within outwards, and in reverse chronological order.

Put simply, this means that the cure is proceeding successfully when the upper bodily symptoms clear before the lower, when more important organs (e.g. the lungs) improve before those of lesser fundamental importance (e.g. the skin), and when old symptoms return briefly, the most recent being first manifest. Although not all these points may be observed in any particular case, the occurrence of inverse responses is regarded as an indication of incorrect therapy. Hence, where the symptoms clear from below upwards, or from the skin to the lungs, or in chronological order of their development, then the treatment is unsatisfactory and not curative.

One thing that is not uncommon in the successful treatment of a chronic disease, is the occurrence of a transient skin rash, even in a patient with no history of skin disorder. This is termed *externalization*, and is usually regarded as a strong indication that the treatment is progressing satisfactorily. Nevertheless, it also indicates that the intensity of the therapy should be reduced (lower potency, less frequent repetition, or a respite from treatment).

Do homoeopathic remedies mix with each other?

In this regard, you must be aware that remedies have certain interrelationships in terms of effect. They may be *complementary*, *antidotal* or *inimical*. A *complementary* remedy either acts synergistically with another remedy, or completes the rectification of physiology commenced by another. An *antidotal* remedy opposes the action of another. An *inimical* remedy reacts with another to produce some undesirable effect (e.g. Mercurius and Silicea, given together or in alternation, may produce eczema). Gibson Miller's *Relationship of Remedies* is a useful and cheap reference booklet in this respect.

In professional work, constitutional and pathological remedies are often combined or alternated, in order to achieve a faster or more profound action. However, this can only be achieved safely and effectively against a knowledge of the interrelationship of the remedies concerned.

In **The Formulary** proper, various mixtures or combinations are occasionally suggested. Obviously, their formulation is such that the components are neither antidotal nor inimical. Unless otherwise indicated, the less experienced should avoid mixing two or more remedies together, except where an acute disease becomes added to a chronic disease. In such a situation, discontinuing therapy for the chronic disease whilst treating the acute may cause problems. Luckily, antidotal and inimical reactions are relatively rare, and only seldom will be encountered. They are even less likely if the remedies are given in *alternation* (e.g. X at 7am and 7pm; Y at 11am and 11pm), except in unusual situations (such as the inimical alternations of Mercury and Silicea, or Phosphorus and Causticum).

Do drugs and remedies mix?

In general, there is no need to interfere with any drug regimes prescribed by the patient's own doctor; unless, of course, they are totally without clinical effect - in which case, common sense determines their abandonment - but, even so, never without consulting him or her. Potentized homoeopathic remedies often work extremely well, even if though the patient is taking drugs (and even in the face of steroid treatment). Perhaps the worst thing that can happen is that the drug will weaken the action of the remedy (which often happens when an antibiotic and a remedy are given together). Remedies seldom interfere with the action of prescribed drugs, and rarely, if ever, appear to react with them to produce inimical reactions. Arnica, however, is one exception, where it sometimes seems to interfere with the onset of local anaesthesia.

Homoeopathic remedies can also be safely given with herbal preparations, nutritional supplements and Bach Flower Remedies. Successful treatment often results from a harmonious medley of a variety of different therapies, developed by the cautious and progressive embellishment of a basic melody.

In which potencies should we initially prescribe and with what frequency of repetition?

The best thing to do initially is to follow the directives of **The Formulary** proper as closely as possible. I have, of course, already mentioned using potencies different from those indicated, and what you should do in the case of a pregnant woman. Always stop the prescription if apparent aggravation or proving occurs.

Although the usual advice is to discontinue any treatment (be it homoeopathic or herbal) for an *acute* illness as soon as the patient is fully recovered, it is better, in my own experience, to continue it for a further 24–48 hours, in order to prevent relapse (except in ultra-acute cases, such as collapse or acute epistaxis). Whilst, at least in theory, clinical proving might result from this prolongation of therapy, in actual practice this is extremely rare, and the advantages of such prolongation outweigh the disadvantages.

Can potentized homoeopathic remedies act locally?

Indeed they can. Thus, Graphites D8 is sometimes added to skin creams for its local effect. They can also be given in the form of sterile aqueous/saline injections for the local treatment of a number of conditions (e.g. carpal tunnel syndrome). There is, however, some clinical evidence that such injectable remedies track from the site of the injection along those routes of two-way ionic/polar molecular flow termed the *acupuncture meridians*.

How do we summarize the differences in use of The Formulary, repertory and materia medica?

In analysing any case, the initial approach is quite different with regard to the three categories of reference work:

1. With **The Formulary** proper, which is a therapeutic index, we begin by selecting a conventional category of disease/syndrome. This is the easiest to use in busy OTC and clinical situations.
2. With a *repertory*, we usually begin by selecting a number of general and mental characteristics, or objective and subjective symptoms.
3. With a *materia medica*, we begin by selecting particular remedies for consideration, based upon personal clinical experience, upon the suggestions of a therapeutic index (such as **The Formulary** proper), or upon the results of repertorization. A standard and comprehensive work of materia medica is thus the ultimate source of information.

What is 'a similior'?

The simillimum may be regarded as a match against symptoms/signs of the 1st degree. A poor match, we might call one of the 3rd degree, and this would be of limited clinical use. Even worse would be a *mismatch* of the 4th degree, produced by 'sticking a pin' in a list of remedies. However, as you will now appreciate, in actual practice, the selection of the simillimum in many instances, and in the *true* sense of the word ('the *most* similar'), may be extremely difficult for the newcomer. Fortunately, nature gives us much leeway and allows us to give remedies of the 2nd degree, which we may term *similiores* (Latin: 'those *more* similar'). The selection of a *similior* often yields perfectly satisfactory clinical results, despite the relative inexactitude of the symptom/sign matching process. In order to expedite the selection of at least a similior (i.e. a remedy of the 1st/2nd degree), **The Formulary** proper utilizes a limited number of alternative, yet straightforward, approaches:

1. A compatible combination or mixture of remedies is suggested, at least one of which is likely to be a similior (or even the simillimum).
2. The adoption of a 'statistical' approach, based upon clinical experience, whereby the remedy most likely to cure the majority of cases (either as the simillimum or a similior) is listed first (and sometimes solely). Where the disease to be treated is of a contagious or infectious nature, this remedy is termed the *genus epidemicus*.
3. The inclusion of mainly symptomatic information in {brackets} after the remedy, which must be taken into consideration for the remedy to be considered as a possible similior. The bracketed statement '{in general}' implies that this remedy is usually the first to be tried.
4. Various combinations of these approaches.

Many of the pitfalls of homoeopathic prescribing can be avoided by following the directives of **A Quick Guide to the Use of the Formulary**, which constitutes Part one of this book.

Further reading

Apart from the books already specifically mentioned in this Section, there are many other excellent ones on this subject available from homoeopathic suppliers. Most provide book lists (see Appendix 4 of Part Four).

Section 4

Bach Flower Remedies

The Bach Flower Remedies have become an extremely popular form of treatment. They were discovered by the Englishman Dr. Edward Bach (1886–1936) in the 1920s and 1930s (Bach is pronounced 'Batch', not 'Bakh', as in German). Their discovery, like all the revolutionary profundities of modern physics and chemistry, was apparently intuitive.

There has always been some controversy concerning the relationship of these Bach remedies to those of homoeopathy. In fact, although they are prescribed in a different manner, they too would seem to rely on water-memory, and thus must be considered as belonging to the same therapeutic group; the physics of this matter being discussed in Appendix 3 of Part Four. Despite these similarities, Bach Flower Remedies appear to mix well with homoeopathic remedies in general, as they do with each other, nutritional supplements, herbal preparations and orthodox drugs. Neither are they contraindicated in pregnancy or lactation.

Bach Flower Remedies are solely prescribed against *psychological syndromes*. These may be deep facets of the personality, of exogenous or endogenous origin, or more superficial, and often transient, circumstantial disturbances. You will find a great number of entries in **The Formulary** proper to exemplify these points. Where the psychological problem has evolved to the psychosomatic, the prescription of these remedies is sometimes useful as an indirect treatment of the resultant physical disease. There are 37 plant remedies, plus Rescue Remedy (which is a mixture of 5 of the others), plus Rock Water (which is a mineralized spring water). The remedies may be mixed to cover any particular case at hand, but I do not recommend mixing more than 3 (or 4, at a pinch) together. If too many are mixed together in one go, rather as one might blend the components of the luminous spectrum, there will be no 'colour' to the prescription other than 'white'. In other words, the amount of different corrective information which can be handled at one time by the psyche is limited. As a general rule, the more recently developed aspects of the psyche should be treated before those at some depth.

Although Bach Flower Remedies are readily available from homoeopathic suppliers, their mode of preparation is still of some interest. In fact, there are two techniques: the *sun* method and the *boiling* method; both being essentially spagyric in origin. The sun method is chosen for plants that bloom during late spring and summer (when the sun is at its strongest) and for Rock Water, whilst the remainder are subjected to the boiling method. The sun method involves placing the freshly picked blooms in a bowl of pure spring water and exposing them to sunshine for 3 hours (in the case of Rock Water, the special spring water alone is exposed). In the second method, they are boiled uncovered for 30 minutes, then allowed to cool. In both cases, they are then filtered and mixed with an equal volume of 40% alcohol in the form of brandy. These are the Bach *mother tinctures*. To prepare a *stock bottle*, add 2 drops of mother tincture to 30ml of the same proof of brandy. The usual dose taken is 4 drops of the stock solution, irrespective of age, weight or size; and this is taken as read throughout **The Formulary** proper. You may, however, find (as with homoeopathic remedies) that instructions for taking these remedies vary. Nevertheless, since their action from the physical point of view is essentially homoeopathic, dosages, beyond a certain minimum, are largely irrelevant. The best way to take the remedies is directly on the tongue, though some prefer putting the drops in a small glass of water, and then sipping or drinking them. The rules concerning the storage and administration of ordinary homoeopathic remedies should be extended to the Bach Flower group.

Bach Flower Remedies are extremely safe and very free of side-effects. Proving does not seem to occur. However, where Bach Holly is used in connection with sexual or emotional rejection, it is not unknown for restless sleep to occur, whilst the person involved attempts to resolve his/her problem by vivid dreaming. Should this phenomenon persist, the remedy should be discontinued.

Throughout **The Formulary** proper, the indications for each remedy in the indicated psychological syndrome are clearly given, and should be noted carefully. However, since the properties of the Bach Flower Remedies are described in common parlance, their selection is mainly natural and swift. In the case of persons taking Antabuse therapy or those who refuse the internal consumption of alcohol, even in the most minimal amount, a few drops of the remedy should be massaged into the skin over the radial pulse of each wrist. This would appear to be a reasonable approach, especially since the wrists, as with mouth, constitute important 'receptor' zones (see Appendix 3).

Further reading

There are many excellent books on this subject published by C. W. Daniel, 1 Church Path, Saffron Walden, Essex CB10 1JP, England. A book list is available upon request.

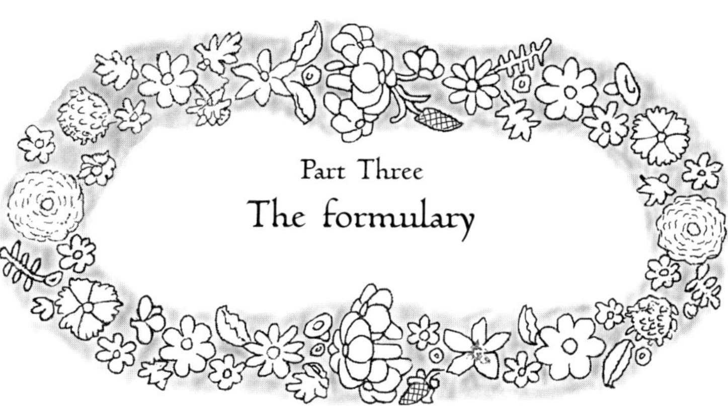

Part Three

The formulary

The icons of the formulary

- Nutritional supplements
- Herbal medicines
- Homoeopathic remedies
- Bach Flower Remedies
- Injections
- Information

The formulary

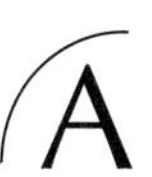

A

Abandoned, fear of being

- ⋇ Bach Mimulus tds.

Abdominal pain

IDIOPATHIC, OF CHILDREN

- ⓘ Wheat or gluten exclusion is sometimes helpful.

OF EARLY PREGNANCY, BENIGN

- ⤫ Cimicifuga racemosa [Actaea racemosa] 30c bd {in general}.
- ⤫ Bellis perennis 30c bd.

Abortion
[MISCARRIAGE]

RECURRENT, PREVENTION OF

- ⤫ Viburnum opulus 6c bd {in general}.
- ⤫ Viburnum prunifolium 6c bd.
- ⓘ It is important to attend to general nutrition, including zinc deficiency (Zinc 15mg om/bd). Caffeine and decaffeinated coffee should be excluded.

THREATENED

- ⤫ Viburnum opulus 30c tds {in general}.
- ⤫ Viburnum prunifolium 30c tds.
- ⓘ Caffeine and decaffeinated coffee consumption should cease.

Abrasion

- ❀ Triple Rose-Water BPC 1934 1 in 2 {cleanser}.
- ❀ Calendula officinalis 5% cream bd.
- ❀ Calendula officinalis 5% ung prn {oral abrasions}.

Abruptness

- ⁕ Bach Impatiens tds {impatient}.
- ⁕ Bach Beech tds {intolerant}.
- ⁕ Bach Vine tds {domineering and inflexible}.

Abscess

BREAST

See: Breast abscess.

DENTAL

- ⚔ Hepar sulph. 6c tds {in general}.
- ⚔ Myristica 30c 45m, three doses only {to reduce severe facial swelling; then proceed to the above}.
- ⓘ The cause must be treated by a dental surgeon.

INCISIONAL

- ⚔ Gunpowder 6c tds.
- ❀ Triple Rose-Water BPC 1934 undiluted {cleanser}.

PILONIDAL

See: Pilonidal sinus and abscess.

Absent-mindedness

ORGANIC

See: Memory.

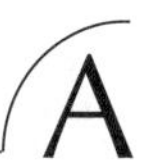

PSYCHOLOGICAL

- ⚹ Bach Clematis tds {day-dreamers}.
- ⚹ Bach Olive tds {due to fatigue}.

Absenteeism

- ⚹ Bach Agrimony tds {shuns confrontation}.
- ⚹ Bach Elm tds {shuns responsibilities}.
- ⚹ Bach Clematis tds {idle day-dreamers}.

Abuse, sexual

- ⚔ Staphisagria 12c bd.
- ⚹ Bach Pine tds {inappropriate feelings of guilt}.
- ⚹ Bach Crab Apple tds {self-disgust; feels soiled}.

Acne vulgaris

- ❀ Smilax spp. 1:5 Ø 30gtt bd/tds.
- ❀ Vitex agnus-castus standardized 10:1 extract 100mg om.
- ⚔ Kali bromatum 6c bd {in general}.
- ⚔ Selenium 6c bd {with many comedones}.
- ⚔ Antimonium tartaricum 6c bd {with much pitting and scarring}.
- 🌶 Zinc 15mg om/bd.
- ⓘ Where long-term antibiotics have been used, treatment for chronic gastrointestinal candidiasis may also be required.

Acromegaly

- ⚔ { Calcarea carbonica 12c + Pitressin 12c + Sulphur 6c } bd.

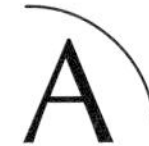

Actinomycosis

⚔ Lapis albus 6c bd {without discharge}.
⚔ Silicea 6c bd {with discharge}.

Addiction

TO DRUGS

✳ Bach Agrimony tds {as an escape from mental torture}.
✳ Bach Centaury tds {weak-willed}.

WITHDRAWAL FROM DRUG

✳ { Bach Walnut +
Bach Chestnut Bud +
Bach Centaury +
Bach Hornbeam } tds.

ⓘ The psychological cause must be treated subsequently.

Adenoids

ⓘ Treat as for tonsillar hypertrophy.

Adhesions

⚔ Thiosinaminum 6c bd {in general}.
⚔ Calcarea fluorica 6c bd {postoperatively, reduction of tendency to produce}.

Adrenal depletion, reversible

❀ Panax ginseng [Ginseng] 1:5 Ø 5ml om.
❀ Siberian Ginseng 1500mg om.
⚔ Kali phos. 30c bd.
ⓘ This may be associated with postviral syndrome, hypothyroidism, severe generalized allergy or any chronic debilitating disease. It may also be caused by

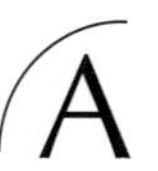

whiplash injury to the neck, bereavement or any other form of psychological shock. Blood cortisol is often normal, but DHEA is usually low (*See* Appendix 1).

Adversity

- ⁂ Bach Oak tds {struggles on against}.
- ⁂ Bach Gorse tds {hopelessness of the sick}.
- ⁂ Bach Gentian tds {easily discouraged by setbacks}.

Advice-seeking, excessive

- ⁂ Bach Cerato tds {requires opinions from many}.

Aerodontalgia

- ⚔ Chamomilla 30c 30m {in general}.
- ⚔ Coffea cruda 30c 30m.

After-pains

See: Labour.

Agoraphobia

- ❀ Hypericum perforatum as hypericin 500μg bd.

AIDS

- Multivitamin-mineral supplement as directed {in general}.
- Moducare® [plant sterols and sterolins 20 mg] 1 cap tds.
- ⚔ Mercurius sol. 6c tds {persistent fever and night sweats}.
- ⚔ Arsenicum album 6c bd {much wasting}.

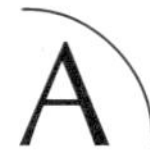

Alcohol, to reduce the craving for

❀ Peuraria lobata [Kudzu] 1:2 Ø 1ml tds.
ⓘ *See also* delirium tremens.

Alcoholism, liver protection in

Vitamin B complex high potency as directed.
❀ Carduus marianus 1:5 Ø 5ml om.
ⓘ *See also* triglycerides.

Allergy

Where the allergen or allergens are known, they be given either singly or in combination in a potency of 6–200c bd, according to response.
ⓘ These isopathics are easily prepared by homoeopathic pharmacists. Where allergies are severe and multiplying, beware of chronic gastrointestinal candidiasis or adrenal depletion. *See also* drug rash, food allergy, hay fever.

Aloofness

Bach Water Violet tds {professionals and intellectuals}.
Bach Beech tds {critical, intolerant and unsympathetic people}.
Bach Vine tds {tyrannical persons, greedy for power}.

Alopecia

AREATA

Vinca minor 6c bd {in general}.
Acidum phosphoricum 30c tds {intellectually stressed young adults}.
Arsenicum album 6c tds {chilly and precise individuals}.

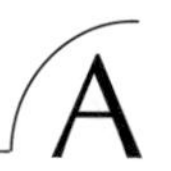

- In some women, adjunctive therapy with Florisene® can also be helpful - see below.

COMMON DIFFUSE FEMALE

[CHRONIC TELOGEN EFFLUVIUM/CTE]

- Florisene® [Vitamin C 24mg + Vitamin B12 3μg + Ferrous glycine sulphate 24mg + L-Lysine 500mg] 1 tab om/bd/tds.
- ✕ Sepia 12c bd {excessive postnatal}.
- Zinc 15mg om/bd.
- ⓘ Iron deficiency, often occult, is the commonest cause. Serum ferritin is a valuable test. *See* Appendix 1. Also watch out for the odd case of occult hypothyroidism.

FEMALE ANDROGENIC

- ❀ Serenoa serrulata 1:5 Ø 30–60gtt bd {by mouth}.
- ❀ Dr Zhao's Fabao 101D™ formula lotion bd {topically, for cases less than 6 years duration}.

MALE PATTERN

- ❀ Dr Zhao's Fabao 101D™ formula lotion bd {topically for cases less than 6 years duration}.
- Zinc 15mg om/bd {helpful in some young males}.

Altitude, ill effects of high

See: Barotrauma; Fear of heights; Mountain sickness.

Altruism, ill effects of

- ⁕ Bach Vervain tds.

Alzheimer's disease

- ❀ Ginkgo biloba 1:5 Ø 2gtt per 6kg body weight bd {halve the dose in those with a past history of stroke or severe hypertension}.

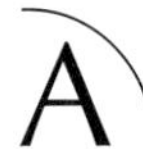

- Inj Vitamin B12 [hydroxocobalamin] 1000μg sc/im once weekly.
- Folic Acid 1600μg om.
- NADH [Nicotinamide Adenine Dinucleotide/Coenzyme 1] 0.14mg per kg body weight om.

Amenorrhoea

- Pulsatilla 6c bd {placid, emotional, thirstless, hot}.
- Cyclamen 6c bd {morose, tearful, fussy, chilly}.
- Senecio aureus 12c bd {cyclical sensation of imminent menses}.
- ⓘ Watch out for intracranial causes and cases associated with anorexia/bulimia nervosa.

Amoebiasis, chronic low-grade

- Grapefruit Seed Extract [GSE] as directed by manufacturer.
- Crataegus oxycanthoides FE 5gtt tds.
- Entamoeba histolytica 30c bd.
- ⓘ Easily confused with IBS or ulcerative colitis!

Amoebic dysentery, acute

See: Dysentery.

Amputation, pain in stump following

- Allium cepa 200c qds {swelling with dull neuralgic pain}.
- Cuprum arsenitum 200c qds {severe burning pains}.
- Borage Oil 1g bd {if diabetes mellitus is present, even though blood sugar is well controlled}.

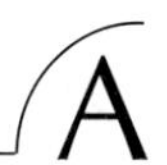

Amyloidosis, cutaneous

❀ Dimethyl Sulphoxide [DMSO] 25–50% gel bd {topical}.

Anaemia, iron deficiency

☙ Iron [as amino-acid chelate] 14mg bd + Vitamin C 100mg bd.

ⓘ All iron supplements must be given with Vitamin C. Iron deficiency often presents without anaemia. *See also* alopecia.

Anaesthesia

ILL EFFECTS OF GENERAL

⚔ Opium 100c 1gt 15m {to encourage arousal}.
⚔ Ipecacuanha 30c 1gt 15m {nausea}.

ILL EFFECTS OF LOCAL

⚔ Chamomilla 30c 10m {anxiety before}.
⚔ Ledum 30c tds {stiffness and discomfort afterwards}.
⚔ Arnica 30c qds {bruising or bruised sensation afterwards}.

Anal fissure

[FISSURA IN ANO]

❀ A cream of the following formulation applied bd/tds:

Non-lanolin base cream	30g
Paeonia officinalis 1:5 Ø	10gtt
Ratanhia 1:5 Ø	10gtt

⚔ Acidum nitricum 6c tds.

ⓘ Treat constipation, if present, as well.

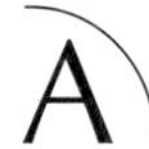

Analgesia

❀ Salix alba FE 1-3ml tds prn {general analgesia}.
⨯ Arnica 200c 5m prn {crushed or trapped digits}.
⨯ Staphisagria 100c 2-4h prn {severe non-specific pain after abdominal operations and deep lacerations in general; after catheterization}.

Anaphylaxis

See: Collapse.

Aneurysm

⨯ Calcarea fluorica 12c tds {to strengthen wall}.

Anger

ⓘ Treat as for irritability.

Angina

ACUTE

⨯ Latrodectus mactans 30c 5m.
⨯ Cactus grandiflorus 30c 5m.

PREVENTION OF

❀ Crataegus oxycanthoides FE 5gtt tds.
➶ Vitamin E 250-650IU om.
➶ Coenzyme Q10 30-60mg tds {not to be stopped abruptly if heart failure is present}.
ⓘ *See also* cholesterol and triglycerides. Any chronic gingivitis and periodontitis should also be treated.

Angioedema

ⓘ Treat as for chronic urticaria.

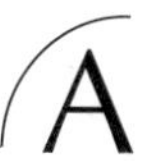

Angular cheilitis

- Vitamin B2 50mg om {most cases}.

Ankles, puffy

See: Fluid retention; Heart failure; Heat oedema; Lymphoedema; Oedema; Varicose veins.

Ankylosing spondylitis

- Calcarea fluorica 12c bd {in general, but especially with aortic insufficiency}.
- Rhus toxicodendron 30c tds {uveitis}.
- ⓘ With aortic insufficiency, *see also* valvular disease of heart.

Anorexia and bulimia nervosa

- Hypericum perforatum as hypericin 500μg bd.
- Zinc 15mg om/bd {anorexia}.
- Bach Flower Remedies, prescribed according to psychological causation, can be valuable; e.g. *see* Bach Holly under irritability.
- ⓘ Some cases may present with amenorrhoea. Male fitness freaks can be anorexic. Some cannot float because of lack of body fat.

Antibiotics, ill effects of

- Crataegus oxycanthoides FE 5gtt tds {diarrhoea}.
- Borax 30-100c tds {thrush}.
- Thuja 6c tds {drug rash}.
- ⓘ Long-term or repeated use of antibiotics may result in chronic gastrointestinal candidiasis, for which special treatment is required.

Anticipatory anxiety, acute or subacute

- ⨯ Argentum nitricum 200c tds {garrulous, restless}.
- ⨯ Gelsemium 100c tds {motionless, silent}.
- ⨯ Aconite 30c 2h {great fear or dread}.
- ⨯ Coffea cruda 100c bd {pleasurable experiences, overexcitement}.

Ants crawling, facial sensation of
[FORMICATION]

- ⓘ Often premonitory of trigeminal neuralgia.

Anxiety and depression, chronic or periodic

- ❀ Hypericum perforatum as hypericin 500μg bd.
- ❀ Griffonia Bean Extract as L-5 hydroxytryptophan 50mg on {reducing to every second or third night, if diurnal drowsiness occurs}.
- ⓘ Bach Flower Remedies, prescribed according to causation, are often valuable; e.g. *see* irritability, apathy. *See also* postnatal depression, SAD.

Apathy

- ⁂ Bach Clematis tds {idle day-dreamers}.
- ⁂ Bach Wild Rose tds {weary fatalists}.
- ⁂ Bach Hornbeam tds {mental fatigue; Monday morning syndrome}.
- ⓘ *See also* chronic fatigue syndrome and exhaustion. Apathy may also be part of a profound depressive illness (*see* anxiety and depression).

Aphrodisiac

- ❀ Jasmine Oil {perfume}.
- ⓘ *See also* diminished libido.

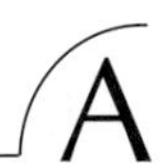

Aphthous ulcers

- ❀ Propolis intraoral 1:1 Ø topically qds prn.
- ⨯ Chrysanthemum parthenium 30c tds.
- ⨯ Sulphur 200c one dose every 4th day {obstinate cases only; may cause exacerbation of concomitant eczema}.
- ➶ L-Lysine 1g tds {short-term dose to clear an attack of ulcers}.
- ⓘ Avoidance of toothpastes containing SLS [sodium lauryl sulphate] is recommended. Iron deficiency, which may be occult, can be contributory; *see* anaemia and Appendix 1. *See also* Behçet's disease or syndrome.

Apnoea

See: Breath holding; Snoring.

Apologetic, excessively

- ✳ Bach Pine tds.

Appendicitis, acute

- ⨯ Iris tenax 30c 1h {only when hospital treatment is unavailable}.

Arc-eye of welders

- ❀ Use eye-drops of the formulation given under conjunctivitis.

Argumentative

- ✳ Bach Chicory tds {totally selfish}.
- ✳ Bach Impatiens tds {very impatient}.
- ✳ Bach Willow tds {ungrateful and resentful}.
- ✳ Bach Vervain tds {over-enthusiastic}.

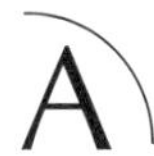

Arrhythmia, cardiac

See: Atrial fibrillation; Premature ventricular beats.

Arrogance

- ☼ Bach Vine tds {domineering and inflexible}.
- ☼ Bach Beech tds {unsympathetically critical}.

Arthritis

DENTAL FOCAL, TEST FOR

See: Focal sepsis.

MENOPAUSAL

- ❀ Zingiber officinalis 1:2 Ø 10gtt tds.
- ➶ Flax Seed Oil 1g bd/tds.
- ✕ Pulsatilla 6c {hot, mild, thirstless, fat intolerant}.
- ✕ Natrum muriaticum 12c bd {hot, thirsty, salt-loving}.
- ⓘ This is a type of inflammatory arthritis that occurs at or just before the menopause, but where tests for rheumatoid arthritis are negative. Reduction of meat and milk products can be advantageous. *See* Appendix 1.

OSTEO-

See: Osteoarthritis.

PSORIATIC

- ❀ Zingiber officinalis 1:2 Ø 10gtt tds.
- ➶ Moducare® [plant sterols 20mg + sterolins 20mg] 1 cap tds for a minimum of 3 months.
- ➶ Flax Seed Oil 1g bd/tds.

RHEUMATOID

- ➶ Moducare® [plant sterols 20mg + sterolins 20mg] 1 cap tds for a minimum of 3 months.

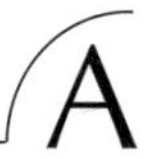

- Flax Seed Oil 1g bd/tds.
- Phosphorus 6c bd {sociable}.
- Pulsatilla 6c bd {shy}.
- Reduction of meat and milk products can be advantageous. Zinc 15mg om/bd may be usefully added in some cases.

Aspergillosis, allergic bronchopulmonary

- Aspergillus spp. 30c bd {in general}.
- Hydrastis 30c bd {intermittent flu-like symptoms, burning in joints, epigastric discomfort}.
- Treatment for asthma or bronchiectasis may also be required.

Asthma, foundation therapy of chronic

- Ginkgo biloba 1:5 Ø 2gtt per 6kg body weight bd {halve the dose in those with a past history of stroke or severe hypertension}.
- Coenzyme Q10 30mg om/bd/tds.
- Extract of Lycopersicon esculentum as lycopene 30mg om {exercise-induced asthma/EIA}.
- Homoeopathic treatment for allergy may also be helpful.
- Acute asthma is best treated with drugs. Effective orthodox treatment must not be stopped abruptly. Buteyko breathing technique is often advantageous. Exclusion of cow's milk products should be tried for at least 1 month.

Atherosclerosis

- Ginkgo biloba 1:5 2gtt per 6kg Ø body weight bd {halve the dose in those with a past history of stroke or severe hypertension}.
- Vitamin E 250–650IU om.
- Flax Seed Oil 1g bd/tds.
- Watch out for undiagnosed hypothyroidism. *See also* cholesterol and triglycerides.

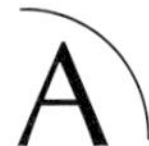

Athlete's foot

- ❀ Neem Oil cream tds.
- ❀ Tea Tree Oil 10% cream tds.
- ✕ Silicea 6c tds.
- ⓘ Resistant cases may also require treatment for chronic gastrointestinal candidiasis.

Athletic support

- Glucosamine sulphate 1g om {to protect joints and tendons}.
- Vitamin-mineral cocktail (daily dosages): Vitamin B2 50mg + Vitamin B6 50mg + Vitamin C 500mg + Vitamin E 250IU + Calcium pantothenate 250mg + Zinc 15–30mg + Magnesium 150mg.
- ✕ Ruta graveolens 200c one hour before exercise {to reduce the likelihood of strain, sprain and hernia}.
- ⓘ Due to depleted iron stores, appropriate supplements are required in up to 80% of women who exercise; *see* alopecia and anaemia. Homoeopathic remedies are not detectable by conventional blood testing. *See also* fitness freaks.

Atrial fibrillation

- ❀ Pycnogenol® [Pine Bark Extract] 20mg bd.
- L-Carnitine 500mg bd.

Attention, lack of

See: Attention deficit-hyperactivity disorder; Inattentiveness.

Attention deficit-hyperactivity disorder [HYPERACTIVITY OF CHILDREN/ADD/ADHD]

- Magnesium 200mg om {average child's dose} for at least 6 months.

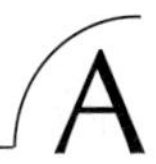

ⓘ Elimination of food additives, salicylates and sugar can be helpful. Some cases require treatment for chronic gastrointestinal candidiasis, especially if they have had many courses of antibiotics.

Autism

⚔ Secretin Co. [Secretin 3c + 6c + 9c + 12c] bd.

ⓘ The strict exclusion of casein and gluten for at least one year may be helpful, and multimineral-vitamin supplements should be provided, including adequate amounts of Calcium and Magnesium.

B

Bacillary dysentery

See: Dysentery.

Backache

See: Lumbago; Sciatica.

Bad

NEWS, ACUTE ILL EFFECTS OF

⚹ Bach Star of Bethlehem tds.

NEWS, CHRONIC ILL EFFECTS OF

See: Bereavement.

VIBES, ILL EFFECTS OF

⚹ Bach Walnut tds.
⨯ Phosphorus 100c bd.

Balanitis

❀ Triple Rose-Water BPC 1934 1 in 2 bd/tds {cleanser}.
⨯ Mercurius solubilis 6c tds {in general}.
⨯ Jacaranda caroba 12c tds.

Baldness

See: Alopecia.

Barber's itch
[SYCOSIS BARBAE]

- ⨯ Rhus toxicodendron 30c bd.
- ❀ Smilax spp. 1:5 Ø 30gtt bd/tds.

Barotrauma, prevention of
[OTALGIA OR SINUS PAIN OF AIRCRAFT DESCENT]

- ⨯ In the morning of the day before departure a single dose of Medorrhinum 200c. Repeat 12h later {2 doses in all}.
- ⨯ Additionally, from morning of day of departure until landing, either Borax 30c or Kali muriaticum 30c 6h.
- ⓘ Don't forget to teach the manoeuvre of Dr. Antonio Maria Valsalva of Bologna (1666–1723).

Bartholin's abscess and cyst

- ⨯ Hepar sulph. 30c tds {early acute phase, to abort abscess formation}.
- ❀ Calendula 1:5 Ø 1 in 20 tds hot gauze soaks {acute phase}.
- ⨯ Hepar sulph. 6c tds {acute phase, where incision is inevitable, to accelerate expulsion of pus}.
- ⨯ Silicea 6c bd for many months {chronic phase, to prevent abscess recurrence or to reduce a cyst}.
- ⓘ Check for venereal infection and treat accordingly.

Basedow's disease

See: Grave's disease.

Bedsore
[DECUBITUS ULCER]

- Vitamin C 500mg bd.
- Zinc 15mg om/bd.
- Cod Liver Oil 1g om.
- ⨯ Carbo vegetabilis 6c bd.

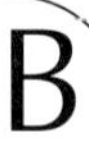

Bed-wetting of children

See: Enuresis.

Behçet's disease or syndrome

- Moducare® [plant sterols 20mg + sterolins 20mg] 1 cap tds.
- Propolis intraoral 1:1 Ø topically qds prn {to oral or genital ulcers}.
- Sulphur 200c once weekly.
- ⓘ Eye complications require the services of an ophthalmic specialist.

Belching, excessive

See: Eructation; Gallstones.

Bell's palsy

- Inj Vitamin B12 [hydroxocobalamin] 1000μg sc/im twice weekly.
- { Aconite 30c + Causticum 30c } tds.
- Borage Oil 1g bd.
- ⓘ The eye should be protected with eye-drops of the formulation given under conjunctivitis. Some cases result from Lyme disease.

Bereavement

- { Bach Star of Bethlehem + Bach Honeysuckle } tds {first month}.
- Bach Honeysuckle tds {thereafter}.
- Hypericum perforatum as hypericin 500μg bd {chronic}.

Big-headedness

See: Arrogance.

Bilharzia, prevention of

- ⨯ Caeruleum methylenum D3 7gtt bd {from 2 days before trip through to 2 days after}.
- ⓘ This treatment is not suitable for those with G-6-PD deficiency/favism. It may be used to reduce the likelihood of topographical reactivation of dormant infection. Routine physical prevention must not be ignored.

Bitchiness

- ⁜ Bach Beech tds {intolerant}.
- ⁜ Bach Holly tds {envy, jealousy, hatred}.
- ⁜ Bach Chicory tds {selfish, possessive}.

Bites

AND STINGS OF INSECTS

- ❀ Glycyrrhiza glabra FE 1h {topically}.
- ⨯ Ledum 30c 15m initially to qds {in general}.
- ⨯ Cantharis 30c 15m initially to qds {midge, gnat, punkie, no-see-um}.

PREVENTION OF MOSQUITO

- ❀ Citronella Oil 4h {topically}.
- ➶ Vitamin B1 50mg bd.

PREVENTION OF SEVERE REACTION TO MOSQUITO

- ⨯ Ledum 200c om {from 3 days prior to exposure and for its duration}.

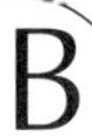

Bitterness

- Bach Chicory tds {if not given constant attention}.
- Bach Willow tds {resentful, nothing pleases}.
- Bach Holly tds {through rejection or jealousy}.

Black eye

- Ledum 30c tds {in general}.
- Symphytum 30c 1h {with pain in eyeball}.

Blemishes, preoccupation with superficial

- Bach Crab Apple tds.

Blepharitis, chronic

- Methyl Sulphonyl Methane [MSM/organic sulphur] 1g bd/tds.
- Smilax spp. 1:5 Ø 30gtt bd {by mouth, not in the eye!}.
- Clemetis erecta 6c bd.

Blepharospasm

ⓘ Best treated according to psychological causation or with general measures for anxiety.

Blisters, common traumatic

- Calendula officinalis 5% cream tds.

Blood pressure

CHRONIC LOW

See: Hypotension.

HIGH

See: Hypertension.

Boils

ACUTE

- ⚔ Pulvis gunnorum [Gunpowder] 6c tds {in general, at any stage}.
- ⚔ Myristica 30c 2h {where there is much surrounding oedema, then changing to the above when reducing}.
- ❀ Echinacea angustifolia FE 20gtt tds.

RECURRENT

- ⚔ Anthracinum 200c om three consecutive days {at outset, then followed by Pulvis gunnorum as given below}.
- ⚔ Pulvis gunnorum [Gunpowder] 6c bd {for many months}.
- ➶ Zinc 15mg om/bd {for many months}.
- ❀ Echinacea angustifolia FE 20gtt om {for many months}.

Boredom, prone to

- ✳ Bach Impatiens tds {impatient for things to happen}.
- ✳ Bach Wild Oat tds {from indecision about correct path in life}.
- ✳ Bach Clematis tds {idle day-dreamers}.

Bossiness

- ✳ Bach Impatiens tds {impatient}.
- ✳ Bach Vine tds {domineering}.
- ✳ Bach Beech tds {intolerant}.
- ✳ Bach Chicory tds {attention-seeking}.
- ✳ Bach Vervain tds {fussy}.

Breakdown, on verge of a nervous

※ Bach Cherry Plum tds.

Breast

ABSCESS

⨯ Phytolacca decandra 30c qds {in general}.
⨯ Silicea 6c tds {after inflammation has diminished, to speed resolution}.

CYST, BENIGN

See: Fibrocystic disease.

FEEDING

See: Lactation; Nipples.

IMPLANTS

See: Foreign bodies.

Breath

BAD

See: Halitosis.

HOLDING ATTACKS, INFANTILE

ⓘ Treat as for temper tantrums.

Breech presentation, medicinal version of

⨯ Pulsatilla M a single dose.
ⓘ The key acupoint for version is Bladder 67 on the outside of the 5th toe.

Brittle nails, common

See: Nail(s).

Bronchiectasis

⚔ { Pulsatilla 6c +
Silicea 12c } bd.

ⓘ Exclusion of cow's milk products can be useful.

Bronchitis

ACUTE

⚔ { Antimonium tartaricum 6c +
Oscillococcinum 200c } tds/qds {in general}.

⚔ Ammonium carbonicum 30c tds {especially with influenza, where Echinacea FE should also be given}.

⚔ Tuberculinum Aviaire 30c om three doses only {stubborn cases}.

❀ Tussilago farfara folia as Schoenenberger Plant Juice [pyrrolizidine alkaloid-free] 10ml bd.

CHRONIC

⚔ { Antimonium tartaricum 6c +
Oscillococcinum 200c } bd/tds.

❀ Ginkgo biloba 1:5 Ø 2gtt per 6kg body weight bd {halve the dose in those with a past history of stroke or severe hypertension}.

Methyl Sulphonyl Methane [MSM/organic sulphur] 1g bd.

ⓘ Exclusion of cow's milk products can be useful. Measures for the prevention of colds and influenza should also be considered.

Bronchopneumonia

See: Pneumonia.

Brucellosis

⨯ Brucella abortus et melitensis 30c once weekly {all cases, in addition to other indicated remedies}.
⨯ Lycopodium 12c tds {late afternoon fever with sour sweat}.
⨯ Pulsatilla 12c tds {orchitis or epididymitis}.

Bruise, common

⨯ Arnica 30c tds/qds.
❀ Arnica montana 1:10 Ø tds {topically only and not to broken skin}.
ⓘ Homoeopathic Arnica may interfere with the development of local anaesthesia. *See also* black eye and capillary fragility.

Bruxism and bruxomania

ⓘ Should be treated for psychological causation or along more general lines for anxiety and depression.

Bulimia

See: Anorexia and bulimia nervosa.

Bunion

❀ A cream of the following formulation [PZ Cream] should be applied tds {must not come into contact with the eyes and hands must be washed carefully after use}:

Non-lanolin base cream	500g
Propolis 1:1 Ø	7ml
Arnica montana 1:10 Ø	7ml
Rhus toxicodendron 1:5 Ø	7ml
Zingiber officinalis 1:2 Ø	7ml
Capsicum minimum 1:3 Ø	7ml

⨯ Perna canaliculus D6 tds.

Burdened, over-

- ⚹ Bach Elm tds {with responsibility}.
- ⚹ Bach Oak tds {with work-load imposed by others}.
- ⚹ Bach Vervain {with work-load imposed by self}.

Burning

FOOT SYNDROME

- Calcium pantothenate 250mg bd.
- Inj Vitamin B12 [hydroxocobalamin] 1000μg sc/im once weekly.
- Borage Oil 1g bd.

MOUTH SYNDROME

- Inj Vitamin B12 [hydroxocobalamin] 1000μg sc/im once weekly {many cases}.

Burns and scalds

- Vitamin E, topical application of the oily contents of any capsule 15m initially to tds.
- ❀ Aloë vera gel, used similarly.

Bursitis

- Inj Vitamin B12 [hydroxocobalamin] 1000μg sc/im once weekly {in arm or buttock}.
- ⚔ Sticta pulmonaria 6c tds {in general}.
- ⚔ Apis mellifica 6c tds {acute cases}.
- ⚔ Kali iodatum 6c bd {chronic cases}.

Calculi

BILIARY

See: Gallstones.

RENAL, PREVENTION OF

❀ Zea mays 1:5 Ø 20gtt om/bd.
ⓘ Soft water is preferable to hard. Meat intake should be reduced. Dehydration must be avoided. *See also* renal colic.

SALIVARY

See: Salivary calculi.

Calculus, dental, reduction of
[TARTAR]

✕ Fragaria 6c bd {in general}.
✕ Calcarea renalis 6c bd.
ⓘ Scrupulous oral hygiene is essential.

Callus calcis
[HARD AND CRACKED SKIN OF THE HEEL]

❀ Aloë vera gel tds {topically}.
❀ Berberis aquifolium FE bd {topically}.
❀ Smilax spp. 1:5 Ø 30gtt bd {by mouth}.
✕ Antimonium crudum 6c bd.

Cancer support

➶ Moducare® [plant sterols 20mg + sterolins 20mg] one cap tds.

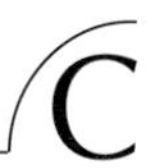

- Methyl Sulphonyl Methane [MSM/organic sulphur] 1g bd.
- Flax Seed Oil 1g tds.
- ❀ Echinacea angustifolia FE 20gtt tds.

Candidiasis

ACUTE

See: Antibiotics; Thrush.

CHRONIC GASTROINTESTINAL

- ❀ Cinnamomum zeylanicum 1:5 Ø 2.5–5ml tds {in severe cases, the lower dose should be selected for 2 weeks to moderate the release of toxins}.
- Caprylic Acid 680mg om/bd/tds {in severe cases, the dose should be increased in stages to the maximum over 3 weeks to moderate the release of toxins}.
- ⚔ Candida albicans 30c om.
- ⓘ Diet is important: the exclusion of sugars and the restriction of fruit, fruit juices, wheat and cow's milk products. *See also* Appendix 1.

Capillary fragility

- ❀ Pycnogenol® [Pine Bark Extract] 20mg om/bd.
- Colladeen® [Anthocyanadin Complex] 80mg om/bd.

Carbuncle

- ⚔ Tarentula cubensis 30c tds.
- ❀ Echinacea angustifolia FE 20gtt tds.

Cardiac failure, congestive

See: Heart failure.

Carelessness

- ☼ Bach Impatiens tds {from impatience}.
- ☼ Bach Olive tds {from fatigue}.
- ☼ Bach Clematis {from boredom}.

Carpal tunnel syndrome

- Vitamin B6 tds.
- Glucosamine sulphate 1g om/bd.
- ❀ PZ Cream [see under bunion] tds over transverse carpal ligament.
- Inj Ruta graveolens 200c once weekly. The site of injection is on the anterior surface of the wrist at the mid-point of the distal transverse crease. The needle should be inserted at an angle of about 30 degrees, with the tip pointing distally towards the middle of the palm. The depth of insertion is about 0.75cm, with 0.5-1ml of the remedy then being injected between the skin and the transverse carpal ligament. It must not be injected into the ligament itself, nor into the carpal tunnel {stubborn cases}.
- ⓘ Watch out for undiagnosed hypothyroidism in bilateral cases.

Caruncle, urethral

See: Urethral caruncle.

Cat-scratch fever

- ✕ Cat-scratch fever 30c bd.

Cataract

- ❀ Eye-drops of the following formulation should be instilled, 1gt per affected eye tds:

Triple Rose-Water BPC 1934	5ml
Cineraria maritima 1:5 Ø	3gtt
Aqua pura	5ml

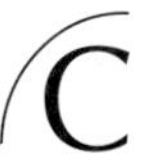

- Vitamin E 400IU daily.
- Colladeen® [Anthocyanadin Complex] 80mg om.
- Cod Liver Oil 1g om.
- ⓘ A diet rich in Vitamin B complex is desirable.

Catarrh

CHRONIC NASAL, OF CHILDREN

- ✕ Pulsatilla 6c bd {hot, placid and thirstless}
- ✕ Silicea 6c bd {chilly and diminutive}
- ✕ Sulphur 6c bd {hot, thirsty and bold; may cause exacerbation of concomitant eczema}
- ✕ Medorrhinum 200c once every 2 weeks {catarrh better at the seaside}.
- ⓘ Cow's milk product exclusion is always worth considering, being careful to substitute with other forms of milk products. Otherwise supplementary Calcium and Vitamins A and D may be required.

IN GENERAL

See: Colds; Hay fever; Polypus; Sinusitis.

Catheterization, trauma from

- ✕ Staphisagria 100c 2–4h prn.

Cellulitis, varicose

- Flax Seed Oil 1g bd/tds.
- Colladeen® [Anthocyanadin Complex] 80mg bd.
- ✕ Belladonna 30c tds.
- ⓘ Also treat as for varicose veins.

Chalazion
[MEIBOMIAN CYST]

- ✕ Silicea 12c bd {in general}
- ✕ Thuja 6c bd.

⚔ Staphisagria 6c bd.
ⓘ The selected remedy should be tried initially for 1 month to assess its usefulness. Surgery is often avoidable.

Changes

ILL EFFECTS OF

⁂ Bach Walnut tds {change of circumstances}.

LIKE THE WIND

⁂ Bach Scleranthus tds {fickle personality}.
⁂ Bach Cerato tds {according to the various opinions of others}.

Chaps

❀ Calendula officinalis 5% ung prn {prevention}.
❀ Calendula officinalis 5% cream qds {treatment}.

Cheerfulness, deceptive

⁂ Bach Agrimony tds {hides mental turmoil}.

Chickenpox

❀ Warm, wet compresses of the formula given below should be applied each night after a bath, and the lotion allowed to dry on the skin (under no circumstances must the skin be rubbed by the material used to apply the lotion). This procedure should help to reduce itching and, thus, secondary infection and scarring from scratching. Where the mouth is involved, the same formula may be used as a mouthwash, but with the omission of the Tincture of Rosemary:

Lukewarm water	500ml
Calendula officinalis 1:5 Ø	30gtt
Rosmarinus officinalis 1:5 Ø	30gtt

- ⨯ Antimonium tartaricum 30c in 4h alternation with Rhus toxicodendron 30c.
- ❀ Pycnogenol® [Pine Bark Extract] 0.5mg per kg body weight bd.

Chilblain
[PERNIO]

- ❀ A cream of the following formulation may be applied bd/tds:

Non-lanolin base cream	50g
Tamus communis fructus 1:5 Ø	30gtt

- ⨯ Rhus toxicodendron 30c bd/tds {prevention and treatment}.

Chinese restaurant syndrome
[MONOSODIUM GLUTAMATE/MSG SENSITIVITY]

- Vitamin B6 50mg om for at least 12 weeks {to reduce sensitivity to monosodium glutamate/MSG}.

Chocolate cravings

See: Cravings.

Cholecystitis and cholelithiasis

See: Gallstones.

Cholesterol, high LDL, adjunctive therapy of

- Royal Jelly freeze-dried equivalent to whole 600mg om.
- Vitamin E 250–650IU om {protective}.
- Vitamin C 100mg om {protective}.
- Benecol bread-spread prn.
- Chondroitin sulphate 500mg tds.
- ⓘ Anxiety may aggravate the condition. Stewed, reheated, constantly warmed and instant coffee may contribute. *See also* atherosclerosis and triglycerides.

Chondromalacia patellae

- Glucosamine sulphate 1g bd.

Chordee

See: Peyronie's disease.

Chronic fatigue syndrome
[CFS]

ⓘ There are a variety of common causes for this, and the appropriate entries should be consulted:

1. ME (*see* postviral syndrome).
2. Occult iron deficiency (*see* alopecia, anaemia and Appendix 1).
3. Occult hypothyroidism.
4. Chronic gastrointestinal candidiasis (*see also* Appendix 1).
5. Chronic giardiasis.
6. Non-diabetic/reactive hypoglycaemia.
7. Adrenal depletion (*see also* Appendix 1).
8. Overuse of orthodox drugs, especially those for analgesia and hypertension.
9. Anorexia and bulimia nervosa.
10. Poor general intake of food.
11. The menopause.
12. Sleep apnoea (*see* snoring).
13. 'Common' exhaustion.

Cicatrix

See: Scars

Cirrhosis, hepatic

- ❀ Carduus marianus 1:5 Ø 5ml bd/tds.
- High potency Vitamin B complex as directed.

Clairvoyance, excessive

⚔ Phosphorus 100c bd.

Claustrophobia

❀ Hypericum perforatum as hypericin 500μg bd.

Clumsy child syndrome

See: Dyspraxia.

Coccidynia
[COCCYGALGIA, COCCYGODYNIA, COCCYODYNIA]

⚔ Hypericum 30c tds.
Inj Ruta graveolens 200c 0.5ml sc once weekly {at most tender spot}.

Coeliac disease

Nutritional deficiency is common, even in those on strict gluten exclusion. The most important deficiencies are: calcium, iron, magnesium, zinc, Vitamin A, Vitamin B6, Vitamin D, Vitamin K, folic acid. Supplements are often indicated.
⚔ Gluten 30c bd.
⚔ Bacillinum 30c once weekly.
ⓘ Intolerance of cow's milk or soya products can occur concomitantly. *See* food allergy.

Cold sore

See: Herpes simplex.

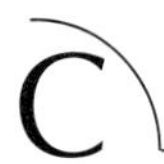

Colds, common

❀ Zingiber officinalis 1:2 Ø 20gtt om {prevention}/tds {treatment}.
⚔ Oscillococcinum 200c om {prevention}/tds {treatment}.
🌶 Zinc 15mg om {prevention}/bd {treatment}.
🌶 Vitamin C 1g om {prevention}/tds {treatment}.
ⓘ Preventative treatment is often usefully combined with that for influenza.

Colic

BILIARY

See: Gallstones.

INFANTILE

⚔ Colocynthis 30c tds {in general}.
⚔ Chamomilla 30c tds.
ⓘ Where babies are breast-fed, the exclusion of cow's milk products from the maternal diet should be tried. Where babies are bottle-fed, switching to a soya milk formula is sometimes helpful.

RENAL

⚔ Berberis vulgaris 30c 2–3h prn {left-sided}.
⚔ Lycopodium 30c 2–3h prn {right-sided}.
ⓘ *See also* calculi (renal).

Collapse

⚔ Carbo vegetabilis 30c 1gt 10m prn.
✳ Bach Rescue Remedy 4gtt 10m prn {often usefully given with above}.

Complaining when ill

✳ Bach Gorse tds {feels all therapy is useless}.
✳ Bach Willow tds {resentful of being so afflicted}.

Concern

EXCESSIVE SELF-

- Bach Rock water tds {introverted self-perfectionists}.
- Bach Heather tds {obsessed with ailments and telling everyone}.
- Bach Willow tds {self-pity and resentment}.
- Bach Chicory tds {selfish and possessive}.

FOR THE WELFARE OF OTHERS, EXCESSIVE

- Bach Red Chestnut tds {fears the worst}.
- Bach Vervain tds {due to sense of injustice}.
- Bach Oak tds {as a matter of duty}.
- Bach Chicory tds {as a means of control}.

Concussion

- Natrum sulphuricum 30c tds {also for post-concussive syndrome}.

Confidence, lack of

- Bach Larch tds {low self-esteem with high ability}.
- Bach Gentian tds {easily discouraged by minor setbacks; useful for discouraged children}.
- Bach Walnut tds {confidence weakened by a dominating person}.
- Bach Centaury tds {timid and servile}.
- Bach Mimulus tds {from fear of the real world}.

Confrontation, enjoys

- Bach Vervain tds {over matters of principle}.
- Bach Vine tds {from domineering inflexibility}.

Conjunctivitis

IN GENERAL

❀ Useful in many cases of both allergic and infective conjunctivitis (acute or chronic), 1gt should be instilled in each affected eye tds/qds {often may be prescribed for several months}:

Triple Rose-Water BPC 1934	5ml
Euphrasia officinalis 1:5 Ø	3gtt
Aqua pura	5ml

✕ Euphrasia 30c tds {in general}.
✕ Argentum nitricum 30c tds {with copious pus}.

SWIMMING-POOL, PREVENTION OF

[CHLORINE CONJUNCTIVITIS]

✕ Chlorinum D8 one dose 1 hour before swimming, one immediately before and one immediately after {three doses in all}.

Constipation, simple

❀ Plantago psyllium seeds 7.5 grams mixed with juice or water bd.
❀ Syrupus Ficorum BPC 1934 7.5ml on or before retiring.
❀ Syrupus Ficorum Compositus BPC 7.5ml on or before retiring.
✕ Opium 6c tds {obstipation - obstinate constipation with no desire to pass motions}.
ⓘ Many cases are relieved by simply increasing the fibre content of the diet and quantity of water consumed each day. Always check the patient is drinking enough. Watch out for cases of undiagnosed hypothyroidism.

Contempt for oneself

⁂ Bach Crab Apple tds {self-disgust}.
⁂ Bach Pine tds {self-blame}.

Contusion

See: Bruise.

Convalescence

- ⋇ Bach Gorse tds {despairs of getting better}.
- ⋇ Bach Mustard tds {non-specific depression during}.
- ⋇ Bach Hornbeam tds {doubts strength to recover}.
- ⋇ Bach Olive tds {lack of vitality due to prolonged illness}.

Corn

- ❀ Calendula officinalis 5% cream tds.

Corneal

ABRASION

- ⓘ Treat as for conjunctivitis.

ULCER

- ❀ Eye-drops of the formula and dosage given under conjunctivitis.
- ❀ Echinacea angustifolia FE 20gtt tds {by mouth!}.
- ⚔ Hepar sulph. 30c tds {with pus formation}.
- ⚔ Mercurius corrosivus 6c tds {without pus formation}.

Coronary arterial disease

See: Angina; Cholesterol; Heart; Triglycerides.

Cosmetic surgery, obsessed with having

- ⋇ Bach Crab Apple tds.

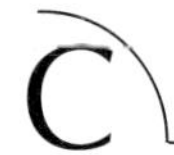

Cough

COMMON DRY

- ⚔ Bryonia 30c tds/qds.
- ❀ Tussilago farfara folia as Schoenenberger Plant Juice [pyrrolizidine alkaloid-free] 10ml bd.

COMMON LOOSE

See: Bronchitis.

Crabs
[PEDICULOSIS PUBIS]

- ⓘ Treat as for head-lice.

Cradle cap

- ❀ The following formulation may be applied bd:

Virgin olive oil	10ml
Tea tree oil	20gtt

Cramp, common nocturnal

- ⚔ Cuprum metallicum 100c bd.
- ⓘ An increase in salt intake is sometimes helpful.

Cravings, to reduce

- ➶ Chromium 200μg om {sweet things in general}.
- ➶ Zinc 15mg bd {chocolate}.
- ⓘ *See also* non-diabetic/reactive hypoglycaemia.

Criticism

EXCESSIVE, OF OTHERS

- ⁂ Bach Beech tds {generally intolerant and over-organized}.
- ⁂ Bach Vine tds {power freaks}.
- ⁂ Bach Chicory tds {possessive and selfish personality}.
- ⁂ Bach Vervain tds {due to high principles}.

EXCESSIVE, OF SELF

- ⁂ Bach Pine tds {exaggerated sense of guilt}.
- ⁂ Bach Rock Water tds {self-perfectionism}.
- ⁂ Bach Crab Apple tds {self-disgust}.

SENSITIVITY TO

- ⁂ Bach Chicory tds {easily feels rejected}.
- ⁂ Bach Vervain tds {offended by opposition to pet causes}.
- ⁂ Bach Willow tds {resentful of most things}.
- ⁂ Bach Vine tds {enraged by opposition to own authority}.

Crohn's disease

- ❀ Crataegus oxycanthoides FE 5gtt tds.
- ⨯ Lycopodium 12c bd.
- A cocktail of supplements: Zinc 15mg bd + Folic Acid 800μg om + Vitamin B12 1000μg om + Cod Liver Oil 1g om + Flax Seed Oil 1g om/bd. Iron supplementation with Vitamin C is often required; *see* anaemia.
- Digestive enzymes as directed at the commencement of each meal.
- ⓘ A reduction of a variety of foods may be helpful, viz. sugar (including honey), meat, animal fat, dairy products (especially cheese) and yeast. Wheat exclusion or reduction may also be effective in some cases. Fish (especially the oily type) is to be encouraged along with a reasonable (though not excessive) intake of fruit and vegetables.

Croup, infantile

⨯ The following three remedies should be given separately 10m in the specified order, repeating the sequence prn {liquid potencies, powders or pulverized pills are to be used}:

1. Aconite 30c.
2. Hepar sulph. 30c.
3. Spongia tosta 30c.

Cut

ⓘ Treat as for abrasion.

Cyst

Bartholin's

See: Bartholin's abscess and cyst.

Breast, benign

See: Fibrocystic disease.

Dental

⨯ Hecla lava 6c bd.

Meibomian, of eyelid

See: Chalazion.

Mucous retention cyst

See: Mucocele; Ranula.

Ovarian, benign

⨯ Sepia 12c bd {in general}.
⨯ Silicea 6c bd.
ⓘ *See also* polycystic ovary syndrome, for which different treatment is usually required.

THYROID, BENIGN

⨯ Calcarea fluorica 12c bd.

Cystic fibrosis

⨯ { Pulsatilla 6c + Silicea 12c } bd {in general}.
⨯ Medorrhinum 200c one dose every 2 weeks.
ⓘ Provision of digestive enzymes is, of course, essential.

Cystitis

ACUTE

⨯ Cantharis 30c 1h-tds {severe pain before, during and after urination, with only small amounts passed each time}.
⨯ Mercurius corrosivus 6c 1h-tds.
❀ Zea mays 1:5 Ø 20gtt tds.
❀ Barosma betulina 1:5 Ø 20gtt tds.
ⓘ Acid fruits and fruit juices should be avoided. A good intake of soft water is recommended. Cranberry juice, barley, parsley and asparagus are beneficial.

RECURRENT AND CHRONIC INTERSTITIAL

❀ { Zea mays 1:5 Ø + Barosma betulina 1:5 Ø } 40gtt tds.
❀ Agropyron repens 1:5 Ø 5ml tds {particularly with urinary reflux}.
⨯ Staphisagria 100c bd/tds.
ⓘ It is frequently necessary to give any of the above for many months. In many cases there is an association with chronic gastrointestinal candidiasis, which must also be treated. Some cases are associated with endometriosis, and adjunctive therapy is required.

D

Dandruff
[PITYRIASIS CAPITIS]

- Kérastase Système Détox Shampooing Antipelliculaire - Cheveux secs {daily shampoo}.
- ⓘ Many shampoos are causative of this condition.

Deafness, chronic

See: Ménière's disease; Otitis media; Otosclerosis; Presbycusis; Tinnitus.

Decisions, inability to make

- Bach Scleranthus tds {generally sways back and forth}.
- Bach Wild Oat tds {concerning correct path in life}.
- Bach Cerato tds {takes too many differing opinions from others}.

Delegate, inability to

- Bach Impatiens tds {feels others are inefficient}.
- Bach Vervain tds {love of overwork}.
- Bach Oak tds {exaggerated sense of responsibility}.
- Bach Vine tds {to retain absolute control}.

Delirium tremens

- Stramonium 30c 1h prn {violent delirium}.
- Hyoscyamus 30c 1h prn {with sexual excitation}.
- Lachesis 30c 1h prn {with great loquacity}.
- Phosphorus 30c 1h prn {with all the above features}.

Delusions of grandeur

- ☼ Bach Rock Water tds {feels others should be of equal standard}.
- ☼ Bach Vervain tds {as a supreme champion of a cause}.
- ☼ Bach Chicory tds {feels able to control all others}.

Dementia, senile

- ⓘ Treat as for Alzheimer's disease.

Dengue

- ✕ Eupatorium perfoliatum 6c or Bryonia 6c in 1h alternation with Rhus toxicodendron 6c {phase of severe bone pains}.

Dependability, utter

- ☼ Bach Oak tds {and hides fatigue}.

Depressive illness

- ⓘ Treat as for anxiety and depression. *See also* postnatal depression, SAD.

Dermatitis

COMMON

See: Eczema; Seborrhoeic dermatitis.

HERPETIFORMIS

- ✕ Bacillinum 30c once weekly.
- ⓘ Gluten exclusion is important.

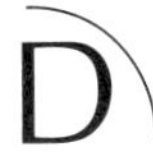

Despair, utter

- Bach Sweet Chestnut qds {distraught}.
- Bach Cherry Plum qds {thoughts of suicide}.

Dhobi's itch
[TINEA CRURIS]

- Neem Oil cream bd.
- A cream of the following formulation bd:

Non-lanolin base cream	30g
Tea Tree Oil	20gtt
Stellaria media 1: 5 Ø	5gtt
Viola tricolor 1:5 Ø	5gtt

- Arsenicum iodatum 6c bd.
- ⓘ Persistent cases may suggest that additional treatment for chronic gastrointestinal candidiasis is warranted (*see also* Appendix 1).

Diabetes mellitus

ADJUNCTIVE THERAPY OF

- Syzygium jambolanum 1:5 Ø 3-5gtt om {Type 2 diabetes}.
- Gymnema sylvestre leaf extract 400mg or 2-4g leaf powder om {Types 1 and 2}.
- Panax ginseng [Ginseng] Extract 200mg om {Type 2}.

NUTRITIONAL SUPPORT IN

- Vitamin E 400IU bd {all cases}.
- A cocktail of: Vitamin C 1g om/bd/tds; Vitamin B12 500-1000μg om; Magnesium 150mg bd {caution in those with renal impairment}; Coenzyme Q10 30-60mg om {not to be stopped abruptly in those with heart failure}; Borage Oil 1g om.
- ⓘ A low sugar, high fibre diet is obviously recommended. High fibre supplements can also be helpful: oat bran, psyllium, guar gum, glucomannan, pectin, and powdered fenugreek [*methi*] seeds

30–90g daily. Fish oils and flax seed oils should be avoided. Milk and milk products are probably best avoided in Type 1 at any age, with precautions being taken to supply missing Calcium and appropriate Vitamins. Reduction of obesity is important.

Diabetic

NEUROPATHY

- Borage Oil 1g bd.
- ⓘ May be prevented by correct nutritional support in diabetes mellitus.

RETINOPATHY

- Colladeen® [Anthocyanadin Complex] 80mg om/bd.
- ❀ Ginkgo biloba 1:5 2gtt per 6kg Ø body weight bd {halve the dose in those with a past history of stroke or severe hypertension}.
- ⓘ Following the advice as given under nutritional support in diabetes mellitus may be helpful in prevention.

ULCERATION

- ❀ Syzygium jambolanum 1:5 Ø 3–5gtt om {by mouth}.
- ⓘ *See also* nutritional support in diabetes mellitus.

Diarrhoea

FAT OR OIL INDUCED

- ✕ Pulsatilla 6c 2h.

RECTAL PROLAPSE WITH

- ⓘ Treat as for rectal prolapse.

SOUR-SMELLING OF CHILDREN

- ✕ Rheum palmatum 6c tds.
- ⓘ Replacement of water and electrolytes is essential.

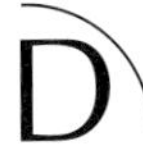

TRAVELLERS', PREVENTION OF

❀ Crataegus oxycanthoides FE 5gtt tds from 1 day before to 7 days after trip.
ⓘ Routine avoidances must still be carried out.

TRAVELLERS' WATERY, TREATMENT OF

❀ Crataegus oxycanthoides FE 10gtt tds.
✕ Arsenicum album 6c 2h {with or without nausea or vomiting}.
✕ Podophyllum 6c 2h {if Arsenicum fails in 24 hours}.
✕ China officinalis 30c tds {to promote recovery after a bout of diarrhoea}.
ⓘ Replacement of water and electrolytes is essential. Persistent cases may require treatment for giardiasis; any lasting for 10–14 days or more are suspicious.

Dictatorial

⁕ Bach Vine tds.

Discipline, excessively rigorous self-

⁕ Bach Rock Water tds.

Discouraged, easily

⁕ Bach Elm tds {by responsibility}.
⁕ Bach Gentian tds {by minor setbacks}.

Disgust of self

⁕ Bach Crab Apple tds.

Disheartenment from minor setbacks

⁕ Bach Gentian tds {negative personality}.

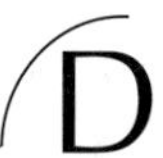

Dislocation, to strengthen after reduction of

- Calcarea fluorica 12c bd.
- Glucosamine sulphate 1g bd.

Dispassionate, utterly

- Bach Wild Rose tds.

Distracted by passing thoughts

- Bach Impatiens tds {of delay by others}.
- Bach Honeysuckle tds {of the past}.
- Bach White Chestnut tds {of worrying circumstances, e.g. litigation}.
- Bach Scleranthus tds {of indecision}.

Distrust, extreme

- Bach Holly tds.

Diverticulitis

- Crataegus oxycanthoides FE 5–10gtt tds {in general}.
- Echinacea angustifolia FE 20gtt tds {to be added in acute cases}.
- ⓘ A high fibre diet is indicated unless diarrhoea is present.

Doormats, timid

- Bach Centaury tds.

Dread

See: Agoraphobia; Anticipatory anxiety; Claustrophobia; Fear.

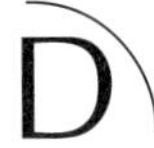

Dreams, terrifying

- ⚹ Bach Rock Rose on {prevention}, 10m prn {treatment on awakening}.
- ⚹ Bach Aspen {if the above fails, with same dosage}.
- ⚹ Bach Rescue Remedy 10m prn {an alternative treatment}.

Drug

ADDICTION

See: Addiction.

RASH

- ⨯ Thuja 30c bd.
- ⓘ The offending drug must be stopped.

Dry socket
[POST-EXTRACTION OSTEITIS]

- ⨯ Ruta graveolens 30c 1-4h prn {in general}.
- ⨯ Hecla lava 30c 2h.
- ❀ A small piece of gauze or cotton-wool soaked in either Plantago major 1:5 Ø or Propolis intraoral 1:1 Ø (or both) can be inserted into the socket, and changed once or twice daily.

Dupuytren's contracture

- ⨯ Calcarea fluorica 12c bd.
- ❀ Dimethyl Sulphoxide [DMSO] 25–50% gel bd {topically}.
- ⓘ The condition may be accelerated by excessive and strenuous use of the hands.

Duty, exaggerated sense of

- ⚹ Bach Oak tds {solid and dependable}.
- ⚹ Bach Vervain tds {passionately pursues causes}.

- ⁂ Bach Rock Water tds {to humanity, by monkish self-sacrifice}.

Dysentery, acute

- ⚔ Phosphorus 6c qds {mild}.
- ⚔ Mercurius corrosivus 6c qds {severe}.

Dyslexia

- Borage Oil up to 2g daily.
- Flax Seed Oil up to 3g daily.

Dysmenorrhoea, functional primary

- ❀ Vitex agnus-castus standardized 10:1 extract 100mg om {throughout whole cycle}.
- Flax Seed Oil 1g tds {throughout whole cycle}.
- Magnesium 150mg tds {throughout whole cycle}.
- ⚔ Colocynthis 30c 1h prn {for cramps}.

Dyspareunia, functional

- ⚔ Staphisagria 12c bd {sexual repression or abuse}
- ⚔ Phosphorus 30c bd.

Dyspepsia, non-ulcer

- ❀ Zingiber officinalis 1:2 Ø 5gtt in 5ml water tds before meals.
- ⓘ This treatment is not always effective when a hiatus hernia is present, and for which a different therapy is often required. Foods and drinks favouring dyspepsia, and which thus should be avoided, include: lettuce, cucumber, tomato skins, fruit skins, fried foods (unless fried in olive oil), coarse wholegrain bread, chilli, oranges (unless tree-ripened), lemon juice, fizzy soft drinks, real ale, dry white wine, champagne. Chiropractic reduction of subluxed mid-thoracic vertebrae can be helpful in stubborn cases.

Dysplasia, cervical, in those 'on the pill'

- A cocktail of: Folic Acid 10mg om + Vitamin B12 200μg om + Cod Liver Oil 1g om {to induce reversal}.

Dyspraxia
[CLUMSY CHILD SYNDROME]

- Borage Oil up to 2g daily.
- Flax Seed Oil up to 3g daily.

Dystrophy, reflex sympathetic

- ❀ Dimethyl Sulphoxide [DMSO] 25–50% gel bd {topically}.

E

Eales' disease

- ❀ Ginkgo biloba 1:5 2gtt per 6kg Ø body weight bd {halve the dose in those with a past history of stroke or severe hypertension}.
- ➹ Colladeen® [Anthocyanadin Complex] 80mg om/bd.

Earache of children

See: Boils; Otitis media; Sore throat.

Ecthyma contagiosum
[ORF]

- ⨯ Acidum nitricum 12c bd {in general}.
- ⨯ Rhus toxicodendron 12c bd.

Eczema
[DERMATITIS]

INTERNAL THERAPY OF

- ➹ Moducare® [plant sterols 20mg + sterolins 20mg] 1 cap tds.
- ➹ Methyl Sulphonyl Methane [MSM/organic sulphur] 1g bd/tds.
- ➹ Flax Seed Oil 1g bd/tds + Borage Oil 1g om/bd.
- Inj Vitamin B12 [hydroxocobalamin] 1000μg sc/im once weekly {stubborn cases}.
- ⓘ Food allergy is an infrequent cause of eczema (wheat, cow's milk or soya products mainly). Nevertheless, artificial colourants and excesses of sugars should be avoided in all cases. Bathing or washing in soft water can be advantageous, since hard water tends to neutralize the antibacterial acidity of the skin. Enzymatic washing powders,

fabric conditioners, perfumes, perfumed soaps and bubble-bath should not be used. Homoeopathic Sulphur is seldom effective these days (however, *see also* varicose eczema). Some female adult cases exhibit hormonal dependence, and remedies such as Sepia 12c bd {in chilly types} or Natrum muriaticum 12c bd {in hot types} may be helpful. A few exhibit exacerbation in the pollen season and isopathic remedies as used for hay fever may be given adjunctively.

TOPICAL THERAPY OF

❀ The following formulation may be used tds/qds and on {in general}:

Non-lanolin base cream	50g
Calendula officinalis 1:5 Ø	10gtt
Matricaria recucita 1:5 Ø	10gtt
Stellaria media 1:5	10gtt

❀ Lavender Oil undiluted bd/tds prn {mild, dry cases}.
❀ Quercus spp. decoction: Boil 30g of any oak bark in 500ml of soft water for 15 minutes, allow to cool, then strain. The liquid should be applied gently with a cloth bd/tds and at night, a new batch being freshly prepared om {infected or weeping eczema}.
❀ Also useful are creams containing extracts of Glycyrrhiza glabra, or a combination of Hamamelis virginiana and pure lecithin [phosphatidyl choline].

Edema

See: Oedema.

Egotism

⁂ Bach Beech tds {hypercritical and prefers own company}.
⁂ Bach Vine tds {power-freak}.
⁂ Bach Vervain tds {tries to influence opinion of others}.

Ehlers–Danlos syndrome

⨯ Calcarea fluorica 12c bd.

Ejaculation, premature

See: Premature ejaculation.

Embitterment

✳ Bach Willow tds {easily embittered by nature}.
✳ Bach Holly tds {embittered by circumstances}.

Emphysema

ⓘ Treat as for chronic bronchitis.

Encephalitis

⨯ Gelsemium 200c tds.

Endometriosis

ⓘ The basic treatment is as for dysmenorrhoea. For urinary symptoms, treat as for cystitis.

Enmity

✳ Bach Holly tds.

Enthusiasm, ill effects of excessive

✳ Bach Vervain tds.

Enuresis, nocturnal, of children

- ⨯ Plantago 30c om in alternation with Equisetum 30c on.
- ❀ Zea mays 1:5 Ø 10gtt on {average child's dose}.
- ⨯ Sulphur 200c once weekly {may aggravate eczema, if present}.

Envy, excessive

- ✳ Bach Willow {grumbling}.
- ✳ Bach Holly 6 tds {overtly angry}.

Epididymitis

- ⨯ Clemetis erecta 12c tds {in general}.
- ⨯ Pulsatilla 6c tds.

Epilepsy, adjunctive therapy in

- ❀ Scutellaria lateriflora FE 5–10gtt tds.
- ❀ Hypericum perforatum as hypericin 500μg bd.
- ⨯ Natrum sulphuricum 30c bd {from a blow to the head, even in the distant past}.
- ⓘ Complementary therapy can reduce the requirements for orthodox medication, and thus reduce side-effects. Hypoglycaemia may be contributory to the onset of seizures.

Epistaxis, common acute

- ⨯ The following two remedies should be given in alternation 10m:

  1. Ferrum phosphoricum 30c.
  2. Aconite 30c.

- ⨯ Ferrum phosphoricum 6c bd {to prevent recurrence}.
- ⓘ Serious causes must be eliminated. Hypertension is often contributory in older persons.

Eructation, excessive, prevention of

⚔ Carbo vegetabilis 30c tds before meals.
ⓘ In some cases, gallstones may be a contributory factor and will require additional therapy.

Erythema

INFECTIOSUM

[FIFTH DISEASE]

⚔ Belladonna 30c tds {in general}.
⚔ Bryonia 30c tds {with arthritis}.

MULTIFORME

⚔ Primula obconica 30c tds.
Inj Vitamin B12 [hydroxocobalamin] 1000μg sc/im once weekly.

NODOSUM

⚔ Apis mell 30c tds {in general}.
⚔ Rhus toxicodendron 30c tds {with arthralgia}.
ⓘ The underlying cause must also be eliminated or treated. It may be caused by drugs (especially the contraceptive pill and sulphonamides), infections or sarcoidosis. It may also be associated with Crohn's disease, ulcerative colitis or lymphoma.

Esophagitis, reflux

See: Hiatus hernia.

Exaggeration about symptoms

✳ Bach Heather tds.

Examination funk

See: Anticipatory anxiety.

Excitement, desire for excessive or risky

⚹ Bach Agrimony tds.

Exhaustion, common

⨯ Kali phosphoricum 6c bd {weariness of mind}.
⨯ Panax ginseng 6c bd {weariness of mind}.
⚹ Bach Hornbeam tds {mental exhaustion}.
⚹ Bach Olive {mental and physical exhaustion}.
ⓘ *See also* chronic fatigue syndrome.

Exophthalmic goitre/goiter

See: Grave's disease.

Extraction, dental, infected socket after

See: Dry socket.

Extroversion, deceptive

⚹ Bach Agrimony tds {conceals mental turmoil thereby}.

Eye

BRUISED

See: Black eye.

DRY

See: Sjögren's syndrome.

STRAIN

⨯ Ruta graveolens 6c tds

Eyelids

CYSTS OF

See: Chalazion.

INFLAMMATION OF

See: Blepharitis.

TWITCHING OF

See: Blepharospasm.

F

Failure

- ⁂ Bach Larch tds {expects failure}.
- ⁂ Bach Mimulus tds {fears failure}.
- ⁂ Bach Pine tds {feels a failure to others}.
- ⁂ Bach Elm tds {failure to cope with responsibility}.

Faint, simple
[VASOVAGAL SYNCOPE]

ⓘ Ammonium carbonate–Lavender smelling salts are valuable, yet often forgotten in view of their antiquity.

Family, over-concern with

- ⁂ Bach Red Chestnut tds {fears the worst might befall them}.
- ⁂ Bach Chicory tds {over-possessive and selfish}.
- ⁂ Bach Oak tds {solidly assists them, even though tired}.

Fatigue

See: Chronic fatigue syndrome; Exhaustion.

Fear

IN GENERAL

- ⁂ Bach Mimulus tds {fear of real things; 'rational' fears}.
- ⁂ Bach Aspen tds {fear of imaginary things; 'irrational' fears}.
- ⁂ Bach Red Chesnut tds {fear for the safety/health of others}.

- ❀ Hypericum perforatum as hypericin 500μg bd {chronic fear}.
- ⓘ *See also* anticipatory anxiety, fright, terror.

OF HEIGHTS

- ✕ Argentum nitricum 200c tds.

Fever

BLISTER

See: Herpes simplex.

INFANTILE

- ✕ The following cocktail of three remedies, dispensed as ABC 30c, may be used as a substitute for paracetamol, being given 1h or so until the fever remits or until a clear-cut picture of the disease evolves:

  { Aconite 30c +
  Belladonna 30c +
  Chamomilla 30c }
- ✕ Where the fever responds but poorly to the above, in order to hasten development of a clear-cut clinical picture, particularly of an exanthem (e.g. measles, rubella, chickenpox), Pulsatilla 30c, a single dose.
- ⓘ Once the diagnosis becomes obvious, treatment should then be directed towards that particular illness.

Fibrocystic disease of breast

- ❀ Vitex agnus-castus standardized 10:1 extract 100mg om {throughout whole cycle}.
- ✒ Evening Primrose Oil 1g om/bd/tds {throughout whole cycle}.
- ✒ Vitamin E 250IU bd {throughout whole cycle}.
- ✕ Phytolacca 30c tds {during episodes of severe tenderness}.
- ⓘ It is important to exclude all caffeine. A low saturated fat diet can be helpful, as can regular exercise.

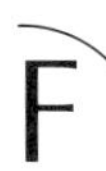

Fibroids, uterine

- ⨯ Aurum muriaticum kalinatum 6c bd {with menorrhagia}.
- ⨯ Aurum muriaticum natronatum 6c bd {without menorrhagia}.
- ⨯ Fraxinus Americana 12c bd {sensation of heaviness in pelvis}.
- ⨯ Sepia 12c bd {overworked, chilly; often usefully given with Fraxinus}.

Fibromyalgia

- Colladeen® [Anthocyanadin Complex] 80mg om/bd.
- ❀ Griffonia Bean Extract as L-5 hydroxytryptophan 50mg on {for insomnia or depression; reducing to every second or third night, if diurnal drowsiness occurs}.
- ⓘ *See* Appendix 1.

Fibrositis

- ❀ Zingiber officinalis 1:2 Ø 10gtt tds.
- ❀ PZ Cream [formula given under bunion] qds.
- ⨯ Cimicifuga racemosa [Actaea racemosa] 30c bd.

Fickleness

- ✳ Bach Scleranthus tds {general indecision}.
- ✳ Bach Wild Oat tds {uncertainty of correct path in life}.
- ✳ Bach Cerato tds {from seeking advice from one and all}.

Fifth disease

See: Erythema infectiosum.

Fingers, crushed or trapped

See: Analgesia.

Fissura in ano

See: Anal fissure.

Fistula

⚔ Silicea 6c tds {in general}.
⚔ Acidum fluoricum 6c tds {bony fistulae}.

Fitness freaks

See: Anorexia and bulimia nervosa; Youthfulness.

Flatulence

ⓘ Treat as for eructation or irritable bowel syndrome.

Flippancy

✳ Bach Impatiens tds {in impatient persons}.
✳ Bach Holly tds {in jealous, suspicious or greedy persons}.

Floaters

See: Muscae volitantes.

Fluid retention, female hormonal

🌶 Vitamin B6 50mg bd.
❀ Urtica dioica 1:5 Ø 5gtt tds.
❀ Vitex agnus-castus standardized 10:1 extract 100mg om.

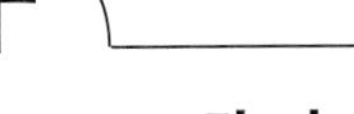

Flushes

See: Menopause; Sweating.

Focal sepsis, dental, testing for

⚔ Hepar sulph. 6c tds {this should be given for a few weeks; should the remote disorder improve, then a dental focus should be vigorously sought and treated}.

Folliculitis

❀ Propolis 1:1 Ø bd {topically}.
ⓘ Barber's itch is a special type which requires different treatment.

Food allergy

L-Glutamine 500–1000mg tds {to reduce permeability of the gut wall}.
⚔ For specific desensitization to foods X, Y, Z... {X 6c + Y 6c + Z 6c...} or higher tds before food (such preparations can be obtained from a homoeopathic pharmacist).
⚔ For general desensitization, Bacillinum 30c once weekly.
ⓘ *See also* chronic gastrointestinal candidiasis.

Foreign bodies

CONJUNCTIVAL, PROMOTION OF REMOVAL OF

⚔ Coccus cacti 30c 10m.

EMBEDDED, PROMOTION OF EXPULSION OF

⚔ Silicea 6c tds.
ⓘ Provided that a foreign body is surrounded by an acute, subacute or chronic inflammatory reaction,

then homoeopathy can be used to hasten its expulsion. In the case of implanted material, there is no risk of rejection provided that there is no such inflammatory response present; in which case, neither dental fillings nor breast implants should end up in the minestrone.

Formication

See: Ants crawling.

Fractious infants

See: Temper tantrums.

Fracture, delayed union or non-union of

- ⚔ Symphytum 6c tds {also to speed normal union}.
- ✒ Magnesium 150mg tds.
- ✒ Zinc 15mg om/bd.

Fright

- ✳ Bach Rescue Remedy 10m prn.
- ⚔ Aconite 200c 10m prn.
- ⓘ *See also* bad news, terror.

Frigidity

See: Abuse; Libido; Sex.

Frostbite

- ⚔ Agaricus muscarius 6c 1h.

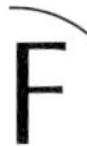

Fury, prone to

- ⁂ Bach Holly tds {from jealousy or hatred}.
- ⁂ Bach Cherry Plum tds {with overt acts of violence}.
- ⁂ Bach Vervain tds {over injustices to others}.
- ⁂ Bach Vine tds {when authority is questioned}.

G

Galactorrhoea, idiopathic

- ⚔ Pulsatilla 6c bd.

Gallstones

- ❀ Carduus marianus 1:5 Ø 5ml om/bd {prevents sludging and should be given even in cases of acute exacerbation}.
- ⚔ Cholesterinum 100c 15m {biliary colic}; 6c bd {long-term treatment of stones and chronic cholecystitis}.
- ⚔ Belladonna 200c 15m {biliary colic}.
- ⚔ Dioscorea villosa 200c 4h {acute cholecystitis}.
- ⓘ A high fluid intake should be maintained - at least six glasses per day - and a low fat/oil diet. Some cases of recurrent pain appear to be related to food allergy (possibly due to intermittent swelling of the biliary ducts). In order of occurrence, these are: eggs, pork, onion, poultry, milk, coffee, citrus fruits, maize, beans and nuts. There is an association between biliary sludging and constipation or obesity.

Ganglion

- Glucosamine sulphate 1g bd.
- ⚔ Ruta graveolens 30c bd.

Garrulousness

- ✳ Bach Impatiens tds {finishes the sentence of a slower person}.
- ✳ Bach Heather tds {about ailments and problems}.
- ✳ Bach Vervain tds {about important projects}.
- ✳ Bach Agrimony tds {to disguise underlying mental problems}.

Gastroenteritis, viral

- ❀ Zingiber officinalis 1:2 Ø 10gtt tds plus Echinacea angustifolia FE 20gtt tds plus Crataegus oxycanthoides FE 5gtt tds {preferably at the same time tds}.
- ⚔ Arsenicum album 6c qds {in general}.
- ⚔ China officinalis 30c tds {in recovery phase}.

German measles
[RUBELLA]

- ⚔ Pulsatilla 6c bd.

Giardiasis

- Inj Vitamin B12 [hydroxocobalamin] 1000μg sc/im once weekly.
- ❀ Crataegus oxycanthoides FE 5gtt tds.
- Zinc 15mg om/bd.
- ① A low fibre, low fat diet with wheat restriction or elimination is to be recommended. Giardiasis is often confused with IBS.

Gilbert's syndome

- SAM [S-adenosylmethionine] 200mg three times daily.
- ❀ Carduus marianus 1:5 Ø 5ml once daily.
- ⚔ Phosphorus 6c twice daily.

Gingivitis

ACUTE NECROTIZING ULCERATIVE

[VINCENT'S STOMATITIS/ANUG/TRENCH MOUTH]

- ⚔ Mercurius solubilis 30c tds {heavily coated tongue}.
- ⚔ Acidum nitricum 30c tds {tongue clean}.

AND PERIODONTITIS, CHRONIC

- Coenzyme Q10 100mg om.
- Citrus Bioflavonoids 1000mg om.
- Coenzyme Q10 toothpaste (Pharma Nord) bd.
- ❀ Commiphora molmol [Myrrh] 1:5 Ø prn {topically to sore or bleeding gums}.
- ⓘ Good oral hygiene and regular scaling are necessary. *See also* dental calculus.

Glandular fever and similar viral illnesses [INFECTIOUS MONONUCLEOSIS]

- Inj Vitamin B12 [hydroxocobalamin] 1000µg sc/im once weekly.
- Glandular fever nosode 30c bd {in general}.
- Acidum phosphoricum 100c bd {additionally}.
- Zinc 15mg om/bd.
- ⓘ Temporary restriction or exclusion of wheat is sometimes helpful. Failure to treat early may result in the development of a postviral syndrome.

Glaucoma, adjunctive therapy in

- Magnesium 150mg tds + Rutin 20mg tds.
- Alpha Lipoic Acid 150mg daily {Vitamin B1 100mg and Biotin 1mg are often recommended along with this}.
- Phosphorus 12c tds {in general}.
- Lycopodium 12c tds {hot people}.
- Silicea 12c tds {chilly people}.

Glomerulonephritis, acute poststreptococcal

- Phosphorus 12c bd {in general}.
- Streptococcinum 6c bd.

Glue ear

See: Otitis media.

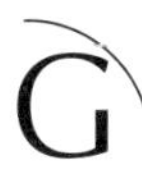

Golfer's elbow

ⓘ Treat as for tennis elbow.

Gout

PREVENTION OF

- One of the best preventatives for gout is the humble cherry. The rules for their intake are: They may be any colour - red, black or yellow; they may be canned or fresh; they must be unpitted, though the stones may be removed immediately prior to consumption or spat out; the stones should not be swallowed; the average 'dose' is 8–10 cherries daily.
- ❀ Urtica dioica or Urtica urens 1:5 Ø 5 drops tds.
- ⓘ Dehydration must be avoided, including that which stems from excesses of alcohol and caffeine. Foods containing purines should be restricted. Red wines, bacon, salami and ham can be 'deadly'.

TREATMENT OF ACUTE

- ❀ Urtica dioica or Urtica urens 1:5 Ø 10gtt tds.
- ❀ Harpagophytum procumbens 1:5 Ø 10ml bd.
- ⨯ Acidum benzoicum 30c tds {in general}.
- ⨯ Pulsatilla 30c tds.

Granuloma annulare

❀ A cream of the following formulation may be applied bd:

Non-lanolin base cream	50g
Echinacea angustifolia FE	30gtt

Grave's disease, adjunctive therapy in
[BASEDOW'S DISEASE]

- Moducare® [plant sterols 20mg + sterolins 20mg] 1 cap tds.

- Thyroidinum 6c bd {in general}.
- Phosphorus 12c bd {sociable}.
- Pulsatilla 6c bd {shy}.

Greed

- Bach Chicory tds {for the possessions of others, love and control}.
- Bach Cerato tds {for advice}.
- Bach Heather tds {for company}.
- Bach Vine tds {for power}.

Grief

See: Bereavement.

Grumbling

- Bach Willow tds.

Guilt

- Bach Pine tds.

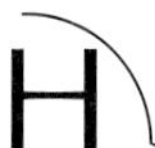

Haemangioma

- ✕ Calcarea fluorica 12c bd.

Haematoma

- ✕ Arnica 30c tds.

Haemorrhage

ADJUNCTIVE TREATMENT OF SURGICAL

- ✕ Arnica 200c 1gt 10m-tds prn {minor cases}.
- ✕ China officinalis 6c + Phosphorus 30c + Ferrum phosphoricum 30c — 1gt 10m prn {profuse and bright red}.
- ✕ Ipecacuanha 30c + Millefolium 30c — 1gt 10m prn {where the above fails}.
- ✕ Lachesis 30c 1gt 15m prn {persistent and dark red}.

PREVENTION OF SURGICAL

- ✕ Arnica 200c 1gt 30 minutes before procedure under general anaesthetic, or after local anaesthesia has taken.

Haemorrhoids

- ✕ Aesculus hippocastanum 6c + Collinsonia canadensis 6c + Hamamelis virginiana 6c — tds {in general}.
- ✕ Calcarea fluorica 12c bd.
- Vitamin E 250IU bd.
- ❀ Hamamelis virginiana suppository 1 om prn.
- ⓘ Treatment of constipation or anxiety may also be necessary.

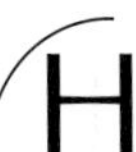

Hair

LOSS, EXCESSIVE

See: Alopecia.

TOO MUCH

See: Hirsutism.

Halitosis

ⓘ It may be caused by consuming pungent foods or by the excessive use of tobacco. Often it results from chronic gingivitis and periodontitis. It may also be associated with Helicobacter pylori infection of the stomach, chronic tonsillitis (cryptitis) and chronic sinusitis. Treatment must be directed accordingly.

Hand, foot and mouth disease

⚔ Antimonium tartaricum 30c in 4h alternation with Rhus toxicodendron 30c.

❀ Propolis intraoral 1:1 Ø topically qds prn {intraoral and dermal lesions}.

Hand-washing, unwarranted preoccupation with

✳ Bach Crab Apple tds.

Hangover

⚔ Nux vomica 30c 2h prn.

Hashimoto's disease

See: Hypothyroidism.

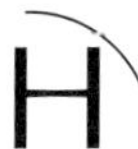

Hatred

- ⚹ Bach Holly tds {overt}.
- ⚹ Bach Willow tds {grumbling resentment}.
- ⚹ Bach Beech tds {from intolerance of the foibles of others}.

Hay fever

- ⚔ Arsenicum album 6c + Sabadilla 30c + Allium cepa 12c + Chromium kali sulphuratum 6c — qds prn {in general}.
- ⚔ Mixed regional pollens 30–200c + Mixed regional grasses 30–200c — qds prn.
- ❀ Ginkgo biloba 1:5 Ø 2gtt per 6kg body weight bd {halve the dose in those with a past history of stroke or severe hypertension}.
- Coenzyme Q10 30mg tds.
- Pantothenic Acid 250mg bd.

Head-lice

- ❀ The formula that follows is applied at night under an occlusive plastic cap for 2 hours; after which the cap is removed, the hair nit-combed, rinsed with 1 cup of cider vinegar diluted with 1 litre of water, and finally and lightly rinsed with warm water; this procedure being followed for three consecutive nights:

Almond Oil	60ml
Neem Oil	5gtt
Eucalyptus Oil	5gtt
Lavender Oil	6gtt

- ❀ Delphinium staphisagria 1:5 Ø applied generously at night for 3–5 consecutive nights, and washed out lightly each morning. After each application the hair must be nit-combed.
- ❀ Picrasma excelsa FE may be used similarly to the above.

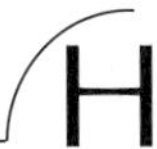

- ❀ After treatment with any of the above, it is wise that nightly shampooing is carried out with any favourite brand to which has been added Neem Oil 15gtt/250ml.
- ⚔ Mezereum 30c bd {only where scalp has purulent scabs}.

Headache, common or garden

- ❀ Salix alba FE 1–3ml tds prn {general analgesia}.
- ⚔ Belladonna 30c 1h prn {throbbing pain in forehead}.
- ⚔ Ferrum metallicum 30c 1h prn {throbbing pain in occiput or in weak and chilly persons}.
- ⚔ Argentum nitricum 30c 1h prn {dull pain in businesspersons or academics}.
- ⓘ *See also* hangover. Chronic or recurrent headaches usually require further investigation to identify any serious cause. Daily headaches may suggest food allergy or non-diabetic/reactive hypoglycaemia. Some cases result from thoracic or cervical subluxation (refer to chiropractor/osteopath), cervical spondylosis or craniomandibular dysfunction (refer to dental surgeon). *See also* migraine.

Healing crisis

- ⓘ This is commonly described as 'getting worse before you get better', and is not an uncommon phenomenon in natural therapy. It can be easily confused with an ineffective treatment in the face of a worsening disorder. The best course of action is to stop the implicated prescription and refer to those with appropriate specialist knowledge.

Heart

ATTACK

See: Collapse.

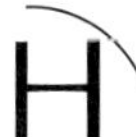

FAILURE, CONGESTIVE

- Coenzyme Q10 30-60mg tds {this prescription should not be stopped abruptly}.

VALVULAR DISEASE OF

- Coenzyme Q10 60mg tds {this prescription should not be stopped abruptly if congestive heart failure is also present}.
- Magnesium 600mg om.
- ⨯ Calcarea fluorica 12c bd {in general}.
- ⨯ Aurum metallicum 30c bd {especially with severe depression}.

Heat

OEDEMA OF ANKLES

- ❀ Urtica urens 1:5 Ø 5gtt tds.

RASH

[HEAT URTICARIA]

- ⓘ Treat as for acute urticaria.

Heel, hard and cracked skin of

See: Callus calcis.

Helicobacter pylori infection

- ❀ Zingiber officinalis 1:2 Ø 5gtt in 5ml water tds before meals.

Hepatitis

ACUTE

- ⨯ Phosphorus 30c bd.
- ❀ Carduus marianus 1:5 Ø 5ml tds.

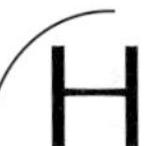

CHRONIC

- ❀ Carduus marianus 1:5 Ø 5ml bd/tds.
- ➶ Phosphatidyl choline [pure lecithin] 1g tds.
- ➶ Shitake Extract [LEM] 1-3g tds.

Hernia

HIATUS

See: Hiatus hernia.

INGUINAL

- ⨯ Nux vomica 30c tds {for minor herniae, or to assist control until surgery is available}.

Herpes

GENITALIS

See below:

SIMPLEX, PREVENTION OF

- ❀ Echinacea angustifolia FE 20gtt om.
- ➶ Zinc Sulphate or Monoglycerate cream once fortnightly {topically}.
- ⨯ Sepia 12c bd {chilly women with monthly attacks}.
- ⨯ Natrum muriaticum 30c bd {hot women with monthly attacks}.

SIMPLEX, TREATMENT OF

- ➶ Zinc Sulphate or Monoglycerate cream bd {topically}.
- ❀ Commiphora molmol [Myrrh] 1:5 Ø tds prn {topically}.
- ➶ Vitamin E, contents of a capsule applied for 15 minutes tds prn {topically}.
- ⨯ Rhus toxicodendron 30c tds.

ZOSTER

See: Shingles; Neuralgia.

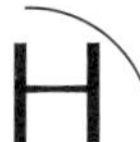

Hiatus hernia

❀ Crataegus oxycanthoides FE 5gtt tds.
ⓘ Chiropractic reduction of subluxed mid-thoracic vertebrae can be helpful in stubborn cases.

Hiccoughs/hiccups

⨯ Magnesia phosphorica 30c 10m prn.

High blood pressure

See: Hypertension.

Highly strung

⁕ Bach Impatiens tds {highly impatient}.
⁕ Bach Rock Water tds {self-perfectionistic}.
⁕ Bach Vervain tds {tense over-doers}.
⁕ Bach Aspen tds {irrationally fearful}.

Hirsutism, female

⨯ Pulsatilla 6c bd {lightens and weakens unwanted hair in many women}.
ⓘ *See also* polycystic ovary syndrome.

HIV support

See: AIDS.

Hives

See: Urticaria.

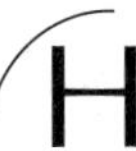

Hoarding

- ✳ Bach Rock Water tds {secretly}.
- ✳ Bach Holly tds {from greed}.
- ✳ Bach Mimulus tds {from fear of running out}.

Hoarseness

See: Laryngitis.

Homesickness

- ✳ Bach Honeysuckle tds.
- ✕ Capsicum 30c bd.

Hopelessness

- ✳ Bach Sweet Chestnut tds {utter despair}.
- ✳ Bach Gorse tds {pessimism}.

Hordeolum

See: Sty.

Hot flushes

See: Menopause.

House-proud, excessively

- ✳ Bach Rock Water tds {self-perfectionism}.
- ✳ Bach Crab Apple tds {obsessed with cleanliness}.
- ✳ Bach Chicory tds {desires to impress}.

Housemaid's knee

See: Bursitis.

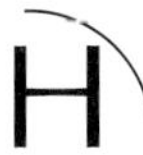

Hurry, everything done in a

- ⋇ Bach Impatiens tds.

Hydrocele

- ✕ Rhododendron 6c bd {in general}.
- ✕ Silicea 6c bd {boys and men}.
- ✕ Abrotanum 6c bd {boys}.

Hygiene, obsessive

- ⋇ Bach Crab Apple tds.

Hyperactivity of children

See: Attention deficit-hyperactivity disorder.

Hypercholesterolaemia

See: Cholesterol.

Hypertension, essential

- Garlic Extract standardized 300–450mg bd.
- Coenzyme Q10 90–100mg om.
- Flax Seed Oil 1g tds.
- Chitosan 5g before food {to oppose effects of a salty meal}.
- ✕ Aconite 100c 10m prn {acute hypertensive crisis}.
- ⓘ A high fruit diet can be beneficial, except in those on potassium-sparing drugs. Those with concomitant migraine may have some form of food allergy contributory to their hypertension. Low salt diets are generally said to be beneficial, but are potentially hazardous to casual visitors to very hot climates. Anxiety is a factor which requires treatment in many cases.

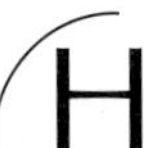

Hyperthyroidism

See: Grave's disease.

Hypertriglyceridaemia

See: Triglycerides.

Hypochondriasis

- ⁂ Bach Heather tds {obsessed with trivial problems}.
- ⁂ Bach Crab Apple tds {from sense of uncleanliness}.

Hypoglycaemia, non-diabetic/reactive

- Chromium 200µg om.
- Magnesium 340mg om.
- ⓘ A low sugar diet should be followed, with frequent savoury or fruit snacks. Exercise tends to improve the condition, and anxiety tends to worsen it. Serious causes, such as pancreatic neoplasm and liver disease may need exclusion. It is sometimes caused by chronic gastrointestinal candidiasis, for which other treatment will be necessary. *See also* Appendix 1.

Hypotension, chronic

- ⨯ Kali phosphoricum 30c bd.
- ⓘ *See also* adrenal depletion.

Hypothyroidism, primary

- ⨯ Thyroidinum 100c bd {in general}.
- ⨯ Sepia 12c bd {in overworked women}.
- Moducare® [plant sterols 20mg + sterolins 20mg] 1 cap tds {Hashimoto's disease}.
- ⓘ Complementary therapies are slow to act and are only suitable as sole initial therapy in the mildest

cases. Otherwise, replacement therapy is indicated, with or without adjunctive alternatives. Although many do well on thyroxine alone, failure of this to control the symptomatology often indicates the need for bivalent therapy with a combination of thyroxine and triiodothyronine (usually best given as Thyroid Extract). Negative thyroid tests in the face of a persuasive symptomatic picture are often misleading and trials of thyroid hormone should be considered. Temperature measurements upon waking are often a valuable contributory means of determining the diagnosis, as is a strong familial history of thyroid dysfunction. No patient can be monitored by routine blood testing alone, and must be assessed on the basis of personal interview. Some cases benefit from the exclusion of goitrogenic foods: brassicas, rapeseed products, cassava, tapioca, sweet potatoes, lima beans, pearl millet, maize. A few are associated with chronic lead toxicity or other forms of chemical poisoning. Iodine deficiency, requiring supplementation, is a relatively rare cause. Sometimes hypothyroidism is associated with reversible adrenal depletion, for which additional therapy may be required.

Hysteria

- Bach Cherry Plum tds {hysterical personality}.
- Bach Rescue Remedy 4gtt 10m prn {acute hysteria}.

I

Ileus, adynamic/paralytic

- ⨯ Opium 30c 4h.
- ⓘ Apart from supportive measures, the cause must also be treated.

Illness, psychological syndromes concerning

- ⁂ Bach Heather tds {describes symptoms in tedious detail}.
- ⁂ Bach Mimulus tds {fear of illness}.
- ⁂ Bach Crab Apple tds {feels unclean as a result of illness}.
- ⁂ Bach Chicory tds {exaggerates symptoms to gain attention}.
- ⁂ Bach Oak tds {frustrated by illness}.
- ⓘ *See also* convalescence.

Immunization, prevention of bad reaction to

- ⨯ Chamomilla 30c one dose 30 minutes before inj and one immediately after {to calm and reduce intensity of pain}.
- ⨯ Thuja 30c bd for 3 days from morning of inj {to reduce local and general reaction, and likelihood of miasmatic disease}.
- ⓘ The above two remedies may be used in conjunction. Thuja does not appear to retard the development of immunity.

Impatience

- ⁂ Bach Impatiens tds.

Impetigo

- ❀ The following formulation may be applied tds:

Non-lanolin base cream	50g
Propolis 1:1 Ø	30gtt
Tea Tree Oil	30gtt

- ⨯ Mezereum 30c tds {in general}.
- ⨯ Antimonium crudum 30c tds.
- ⨯ Antimonium tartaricum 30c tds.

Impetuosity

- ✳ Bach Impatiens tds {from impatience}.
- ✳ Bach Vervain tds {agrees too quickly to take on new tasks}.
- ✳ Bach Cherry Plum tds {out of desperation}.

Implants

See: Foreign bodies.

Impotence

- ❀ Liriosma ovata [Muira Puama] FE 0.5–2ml tds.
- ❀ Ginkgo biloba 1:5 2gtt per 6kg Ø body weight bd {where atherosclerosis is contributory; halve the dose in those with a past history of stroke or severe hypertension}.
- ⨯ Selenium 30c bd {penis relaxes on attempted coition}.

Impudence/rudeness

- ✳ Bach Beech tds {from intolerance of the mistakes of others}.
- ✳ Bach Willow tds {from simmering resentment}.
- ✳ Bach Chicory tds {when attention to self is denied}.

Inattentiveness

- ⚹ Bach White Chestnut tds {preoccupation with a worrying event}.
- ⚹ Bach Clematis tds {day-dreamers}.
- ⚹ Bach Honeysuckle tds {dwells on the past}.
- ⓘ *See also* attention deficit-hyperactivity disorder.

Incontinence

See: Enuresis; Stress incontinence.

Indecision

See: Decisions.

Indifference to the needs of others

- ⚹ Bach Beech tds {intolerance of the mistakes of others}.
- ⚹ Bach Impatiens tds {intolerant of slowness}.
- ⚹ Bach Vine tds {power-freak}.
- ⚹ Bach Chicory tds {demands constant attention}.
- ⚹ Bach Holly tds {from jealousy, envy or hatred}.

Indigestion, common

See: Dyspepsia.

Indignation

- ⚹ Bach Beech tds {over the mistakes of others}.
- ⚹ Bach Chicory tds {over lack of attention from others}.
- ⚹ Bach Vervain tds {over injustices in the world}.

Infertility

MALE

- Zinc 15mg bd.
- Vitamin C 500mg bd.
- Coenzyme Q10 30mg om.
- Vitamin E 250IU om.
- Inj Vitamin B12 [hydroxocobalamin] 1000µg sc/im once weekly.
- ⓘ Excesses of alcohol should be avoided. Much tap-water now contains chemical products with oestrogenic effects of some significance. Only spring water from high, non-industrialized, non-arable areas of low population should be consumed, therefore (e.g. Scottish Highlands, Shropshire Longmynd).

OBSCURE FEMALE

- Vitex agnus-castus standardized 10:1 extract 100mg om.
- Vitamin E 250IU om.
- Multimineral-vitamin supplement as directed.
- ⓘ The following factors favour infertility: being overweight or underweight; smoking; caffeine consumption (decaffeinated coffee may, however, cause spontaneous abortion); poor general nutrition; iron deficiency, which may be occult - *see* anaemia. Gluten sensitivity is an occasional cause, and an indication for exclusion (*see also* food allergy) and often the initial prescription of Folic Acid 5mg tds. *See also* polycystic ovary syndrome.

Influenced by others, ill effects of being

- Bach Walnut tds {from a dominating person}.
- Bach Centaury tds {from being generally weak-willed or servile}.
- Bach Cerato tds {from lack of confidence in own judgment}.
- Bach Red Chestnut tds {fear for the safety/health of others}.
- ⓘ *See also* clairvoyance and manipulated.

Influenza

❀ Echinacea angustifolia FE 20gtt om {prevention}/tds {treatment}.

⤫ Bacillinum 30c + Influenzinum Co. 30c — once monthly {prevention}.

⤫ Nux vomica 30c + Natrum sulphuricum 30c + Magnesia phosphorica 30c + Pyrogen 30c — qds {treatment, in general}.

⤫ Gelsemium 30c qds.

ⓘ Preventative treatment for common colds is often usefully combined with that for influenza. Additional treatment for dry cough or acute bronchitis may be required, according to circumstances. Zinc and Vitamin C supplementation as for common colds can also be useful. Postviral syndrome can result.

Ingrowing toenail

❀ Propolis 1:1 Ø bd {topically}.

⤫ Magnetis polus australis 30c bd.

ⓘ The services of a chiropodist/podiatrist may also be required.

Inquisitive/nosey, excessively

⋇ Bach Vervain tds {from genuine and intense interest}.

⋇ Bach Impatiens tds {from desire to expedite matters}.

⋇ Bach Chicory tds {to gain control by knowing secrets}.

Insensitivity

See: Indifference.

Insomnia, common

❀ Tab { Hops powder 167mg + Valerian powder 250mg } 1-3 tab as single dose on prn.
⨯ Coffea cruda 200c on {from mind full of thoughts}.
❀ Griffonia bean as L-5 hydroxytryptophan 50mg on {reducing to every second or third night, if diurnal drowsiness occurs}.
ⓘ The cause of the insomnia may also require treatment. *See* anxiety and depression.

Intercostal rheumatism

⨯ Ranunculus bulbosus 30c tds.
ⓘ Many improve with chiropractic manipulation of the thoracic spine.

Intermittent claudication

ⓘ Treat as for atherosclerosis.

Intertrigo

ⓘ Treat as for dhobi's itch.

Intimidating

✳ Bach Vine tds.

Intolerance

✳ Bach Beech tds {of mistakes of others}.
✳ Bach Impatiens tds {of slowness of others}.
✳ Bach Rock Water tds {of imprecision in others}.
✳ Bach Vervain tds {of those with different ideas}.

Iritis

ⓘ Treat as for uveitis.

Irritability, excessive

- ⚔ Staphisagria 12c bd {from stifled vexation/suppressed anger}.
- ✳ Bach Impatiens tds {over most things}.
- ✳ Bach Vervain tds {from frustration over injustices}.
- ✳ Bach Holly tds {due to hatred, envy or jealousy}.
- ✳ Bach Willow tds {generally bitter}.
- ✳ Bach Beech tds {over faults of others}.
- ✳ Bach Chicory tds {when attention of others is turned elsewhere}.
- ✳ Bach Cherry Plum tds {prone to acts of violence}.
- ✳ Bach Vine tds {when authority is questioned}.

Irritable bowel syndrome
[IBS]

- ❀ Crataegus oxycanthoides FE 5gtt tds.
- ⚔ Pulsatilla 6c bd {in mild-natured, fat/oil-intolerant persons}.
- ⚔ Lycopodium 12c bd {with lower abdominal distention}.
- ⚔ China officinalis 30c bd {with general abdominal distention}.
- ⓘ A low fibre diet is often indicated, with less brassicas and pulses. IBS is sometimes confused with giardiasis. Beware of the patient whose apparent IBS starts during or within a few months of a trip abroad or after a bout of food poisoning. Some cases of apparent IBS are due to chronic gastrointestinal candidiasis, for which other treatment may be warranted.

Isolation

- Bach Water Violet tds {aloof and detached}.
- Bach Rock Water tds {withdrawn self-perfectionists}.
- Bach Impatiens tds {to escape from irritation caused by others}.
- Bach Heather tds {loathes being alone}.

J

Jaundice

See: Alcoholism; Cirrhosis; Gallstones; Gilbert's syndrome; Hepatitis; Wilson's disease

Jealousy, ill effects of

⁂ Bach Holly tds.

Jellyfish stings

❀ Vinegar should be applied liberally to any adherent tentacles (not alcohol or methylated spirits!).

❀ Once they are removed, a thick paste of papain and water should be rubbed in.

ⓘ In the case of the box jellyfish, stings are potentially lethal, and early vinegar applications may be life-saving. A specific antivenin is available.

Jet lag

⚔ Cocculus indicus 30c 12h from 2 days before flight to 3 days after.

❀ Griffonia bean as L-5 hydroxytryptophan 50mg 24h from 10pm (with watch adjusted to destination time) on the first day of flight to 5 days after arrival {reducing to 48h, if excessive diurnal drowsiness occurs}.

Jokers, deceptive

⁂ Bach Agrimony tds {hides inner turmoil}.

Joy, fear of

⚔ Coffea cruda 100c bd.

K

Kala azar, Mediterranean infantile
[VISCERAL LEISHMANIASIS]

- Arsenicum album 6c tds.

Keen, excessively

- Bach Vervain tds {from general enthusiasm}.
- Bach Impatiens tds {from a desire for swift conclusions}.

Keloid

See: Scars.

Kidney stones

See: Calculi; Colic.

Killers

- Bach Cherry Plum tds {generally prone to sudden violent impulses}.
- Bach Holly tds {*crime passionnel* types}.

Know-it-alls

- Bach Vine tds {domineering and self-opinionated}.
- Bach Beech tds {critical and self-opinionated}.

L

Labour

AFTER-PAINS OF

⨯ Caulophyllum 6c 30m prn.

HOMOEOPATHIC INDUCTION OF

⨯ Caulophyllum 30c 6h.

PREPARATION FOR

⨯ Caulophyllum 30c one dose weekly for 4 weeks before term {encourages cervical dilatation at term}.

Laceration

ⓘ Treat as for abrasion and haemorrhage. *See also* analgesia, wound healing.

Lactation

INADEQUATE

⨯ Pulsatilla 6c bd.
❀ Urtica urens/dioica 1:5 Ø 5gtt tds.

INAPPROPRIATE

See: Galactorrhoea.

TO STOP

⨯ Lac caninum 200c bd {maximum 6 doses}.

Laryngitis

ACUTE

- ⨯ Arum triphyllum 30c tds {in general}.
- ⨯ Argentum metallicum 30c {with pain in larynx}.
- ⓘ Treatment for common colds is also sometimes indicated.

CHRONIC

- ⨯ Arum triphyllum 30c bd {in general}.
- ⨯ Phosphorus 12c bd.
- ⓘ Treatment as for chronic sinusitis may be required instead, if a postnasal drip is present.

Laughter, prone to uncontrollable

- ✳ Bach Cherry Plum tds.

Lax ligament syndrome

- ⨯ Calcarea fluorica 12c bd.
- ⓘ The carrying angle of the elbow is >180°.

Laziness

See: Apathy.

Leaky gut syndrome

See: Food allergy.

Learn

FAILURE TO, FROM PAST MISTAKES

- ✳ Bach Chestnut Bud tds.

FAILURE TO, IN CHILDREN

See: Apathy; Attention deficit-hyperactivity disorder; Autism; Dyslexia.

Lethargy

See: Apathy; Chronic fatigue syndrome; Exhaustion.

Leukoplakia, oral

- Vitamin E 400IU bd.
- Spirulina fusiformis 1g om.

Libido

DIMINISHED

- ❀ Liriosma ovata [Muira Puama] FE 0.5–2ml tds {♂/♀}.
- ⓘ Treatment of any hormonal problems in females is also warranted, as is that of any psychological contributory factor in either sex. *See also* sex.

EXCESSIVE

See: Sex.

Lice

See: Crabs; Head-lice.

Lichen planus

- ⨯ Arsenicum album 12c bd {oral type, in general}.
- ❀ Aloë vera gel tds prn {oral type, topically}.
- ⓘ It is sometimes a manifestation of chronic gastrointestinal candidiasis, for which special treatment is required.

Lips, cracked

AT CORNERS

See: Angular cheilitis.

FROM EXPOSURE

❀ Calendula officinalis 5% ung prn.

Litigation, impending, preys on mind

⁕ Bach White Chestnut tds.

Loners

⁕ Bach Impatiens tds {prefers being alone for thinking or working}.
⁕ Bach Water Violet tds {aloof and enjoys being alone generally}.
⁕ Bach Clematis tds {day-dreamers living in a world of their own}.

Love

ABSENCE OF, WITH SEXUAL FRUSTRATION

✕ Staphisagria 12c bd.

DREAMY OR SOPPY

⁕ Bach Clematis tds.

PASSIONATE AND JEALOUS

⁕ Bach Holly tds.

PAST, DWELLS UPON

⁕ Bach Honeysuckle tds.

POSSESSIVE AND SELFISH

- Bach Chicory tds.

REJECTED OR UNREQUITED PASSIONATE

- Bach Holly tds.

Lumbago

- Glucosamine sulphate 1g bd {chronic; may take up to 3 months before improvement occurs}.
- Inj Ruta graveolens 200c 1ml sc once weekly over each sacroiliac joint {acute/chronic}.
- Salix alba FE 1–3ml tds prn.
- Bellis perennis 30c qds {feels bruised but loosens with continued motion; gardener's/camper's backache}.
- Rhus toxicodendron 30c qds {feels stiff and painful but loosens with continued motion}.
- Arnica 30c qds {feels bruised but worse from continued motion}.
- Calcarea fluorica 6c tds {chronic backache where other measures fail}.
- ⓘ Osteopathic/chiropractic manipulative technique is additionally indicated in most cases. In older adults (usually over 60), beware of multiple myeloma (severe, unremitting lumbago), where the measures given above are likely to fail. *See also* Scheuermann's disease.

Lupus erythematosus, systemic and discoid [SLE/DLE]

See: Systemic and discoid lupus erythematosus.

Lyme disease

PREVENTION OF

- Borrelia burgdorferi 30c once weekly {yet unproven}.

TREATMENT OF

ⓘ Although treatment with antibiotics is strongly indicated, adjunctive therapy with complementary medicines is desirable in the 2nd and 3rd stages, according to the nature of the complication, e.g. Bell's palsy.

Lymphadenopathy, cervical

BENIGN, OF CHILDREN

⚔ Lapis albus 6c bd.

CHRONIC TUBERCULAR, ADJUNCTIVE THERAPY OF

⚔ Bacillinum 100c one dose fortnightly.

Lymphoedema

OF LOWER EXTREMITIES

⚔ Silicea 12c bd {in general}.
⚔ Arsenicum album 12c bd.

POST-MASTECTOMY

❀ Ruscus aculeatus Extract standardized [9-11% ruscogenins] 100mg tds.

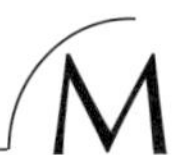

M

Macular degeneration

- ❀ Ginkgo biloba 1:5 2gtt per 6kg Ø body weight bd {halve the dose in those with a past history of stroke or severe hypertension}.
- Colladeen® [Anthocyanadin Complex] 80mg om/bd.

Malaria, adjunctive prevention of

- ⨉ Malaria officinalis 30c bd Monday, plus China officinalis D8 bd Tuesday through to Sunday {this scheme may be repeated for many weeks/months, and should be continued for 6 weeks after quitting the malaria zone}.
- ⓘ *See also* bites, prevention of mosquito - which is undoubtedly even more important!

Malingering

- ⋇ Bach Wild Rose tds {from laziness}.
- ⋇ Bach Elm tds {from wishing to avoid excessive responsibility}.
- ⋇ Bach Olive tds {from exhaustion}.

Manipulated, easily

- ⋇ Bach Centaury tds {servile doormats}.
- ⋇ Bach Agrimony tds {easily driven to hazardous pursuits to hide internal misery or stress}.

Manipulative, highly

- ⋇ Bach Chicory tds.

Mannerisms

- ⋇ Bach Vervain tds {theatrically excessive}.
- ⋇ Bach Beech tds {irritated by those of others}.

Martyrdom

- ⋇ Bach Rock Water tds {to own high ideals and to set an example}.
- ⋇ Bach Vervain tds {to a cause}.

Mastectomy, lymphoedema following

See: Lymphoedema.

Mastoid cavity, chronic infection of

- ⨯ Kali sulphuricum 12c bd.
- ❀ Triple Rose-Water BPC 1934 3gtt tds {topically}.

Maternal, overly

- ⋇ Bach Red Chestnut tds {unselfish concern}.
- ⋇ Bach Chicory tds {possessive}.
- ⋇ Bach Centaury tds {slavish}.

ME
[MYALGIC ENCEPHALOPATHY]

See: Postviral syndrome.

Measles

- ⨯ Pulsatilla 6c 4h.

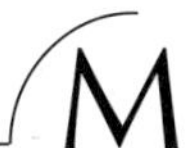

Meddling

- ⁂ Bach Impatiens tds {to hasten others}.
- ⁂ Bach Chicory tds {to manipulate others}.
- ⁂ Bach Vervain tds {to persuade others}.

Meibomian cyst

See: Chalazion.

Memory, poor

- Vitamin B1 100mg om {with obscure causation}.
- Vitamin B6 50mg bd {in women with hormonal problems}.
- ❀ Ginkgo biloba 1:5 2gtt per 6kg Ø body weight bd {in the elderly; halve the dose in those with a past history of stroke or severe hypertension}.
- ⁂ Bach White Chestnut tds {due to mind filled with own problems}.
- ⁂ Bach Vervain tds {due to mind filled with injustices to others}.
- ⁂ Bach Honeysuckle tds {due to constant dwelling on the past}.
- ⓘ *See also* absent-mindedness.

Ménière's disease

- ⨯ Acidum muriaticum 12c bd {in general}.
- ⨯ Natrum salicylicum 30c bd.
- ⨯ Acidum salicylicum 30c bd.
- ⨯ Calcarea carbonica 30c bd.
- ⓘ The above may be tried for 2 weeks at a time in sequence until the best is found. Many cases have a psychological origin, and additional treatment for anxiety is often warranted. Some improve by cutting out refined carbohydrates.

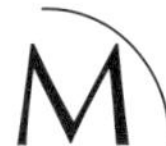

Meningitis, adjunctive therapy of

- ⚔ Cicuta virosa 30c 4h {in general}.
- ⚔ Ammonium carbonicum 30c 4h.
- ⚔ Meningococcinum 6c 4h {meningococcal meningitis, either separately or in combination with either of the above}.

Menopause

ARTHRITIS IN

See: Arthritis.

HOT FLUSHES IN

- ❀ Vitex agnus-castus standardized 10:1 extract 100mg om.
- ➶ Vitamin C 400mg tds plus Hesperidin 400mg tds.
- ➶ Vitamin E 800IU om.
- ➶ Flax Seed Oil 1g tds.
- ⚔ Oestradiol 12c bd.
- ⓘ A diet high in soya products is recommended, as is regular exercise.

Menorrhagia, common

- ❀ Vitex agnus-castus standardized 10:1 extract 100mg om.
- ➶ Vitamin C 200mg tds plus Bioflavonoids 200mg tds.
- ➶ Vitamin A 3000μg om.
- ➶ Vitamin E 250IU om {menorrhagia from IUD}.
- ❀ Cinnamomum zeylanicum 1:5 Ø 2.5–5ml tds.
- ⓘ Any of the above should be taken throughout the cycle. Iron deficiency is both a cause and an effect of menorrhagia, and must be treated, if present (*see* anaemia and Appendix 1). Serious causes, such as Grave's disease, must be eliminated. *See also* fibroids.

Menstrual disorders

See: Amenorrhoea; Dysmenorrhoea; Endometriosis; Fibroids; Menorrhagia.

Mercy, without

- ✳ Bach Holly tds {vengeful and hateful).
- ✳ Bach Vine tds {dictators}.

Meticulous, overly

- ✳ Bach Beech tds {precise}.
- ✳ Bach Vervain tds {fussy but imprecise}.
- ✳ Bach Crab Apple tds {preoccupied with minute detail}.
- ✳ Bach Rock Water tds {preoccupied with self-perfection}.

Midge and gnat bites

See: Bites.

Migraine

PREVENTION OF

- ❀ Feverfew tab/cap as parthenolide 250μg om {Ø is ineffective}.
- ❀ Zingiber officinalis 1:5 Ø 1.5–3ml tds.
- ❀ Ginkgo biloba 1:5 2gtt per 6kg Ø body weight bd {halve the dose in those with a past history of stroke or severe hypertension}.
- 🌶 Flax Seed Oil 1g bd.
- ❀ Salix alba FE 1–3ml om.
- ⓘ Causes include: food allergy, lactose intolerance, cheese, chocolate, red wine, port, instant coffee, hypoglycaemia, anxiety, premenstrual syndrome and problems with the cervical or upper thoracic spine (referral for chiropractic or osteopathic treatment is often helpful). Serious intracranial causes must be eliminated.

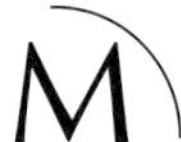

TREATMENT OF ACUTE

- ⨯ Iris versicolor 200c 30m prn {in general}.
- ⨯ Sanguinaria 200c 30m prn {right-sided}.
- ⨯ Spigelia 200c 30m prn {left-sided}.

Migrainous neuralgia

- ⓘ Treat as for migraine.

Misguided

- ✳ Bach Walnut tds {occasionally}.
- ✳ Bach Centaury tds {easily influenced and servile}.
- ✳ Bach Cerato tds {seeks advice from everyone}.

Mistakes

- ✳ Bach Impatiens tds {made from being too hurried}.
- ✳ Bach Chestnut Bud tds {fails to learn from those of the past}.
- ✳ Bach Pine tds {blames self for those of others}.

Molluscum contagiosum

- ❀ A cream of the following formulation should be applied bd:

Non-lanolin base cream	50g
Propolis 1:1 Ø	40gtt

- ⨯ Silicea 12c bd.

Monday morning syndrome

- ✳ Bach Hornbeam 1h prn.
- ⓘ *See also* hangover.

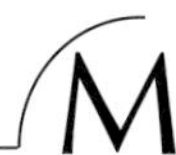

Monge's disease

See: Mountain sickness.

Mononucleosis, infectious

See: Glandular fever.

Moodiness

- ⚹ Bach Scleranthus tds {mood swings}.
- ⚹ Bach Willow tds {grumbling}.
- ⚹ Bach Chicory tds {moany}.

Morning sickness

- ☛ Phytomenadione 5mg on plus Vitamin C 500mg on.
- ☛ Vitamin B6 10–25mg tds.
- ❀ Zingiber officinalis 1:2 Ø 5–10gtt 1–2h prn {max. 50gtt daily}.
- ⓘ The diet should be rich in Vitamin B complex.

Motion sickness

- ☛ Zingiber officinalis 1:2 Ø 5–10gtt 1–2h prn {may also be used preventively by giving 30 minutes before trip}.
- ⨯ { Cocculus indicus 30c + Petroleum 6c + Tabacum 6c } 2–4h prn {also may be used preventively as above}.

Mountain sickness

ACUTE

- ⨯ Coca 30c tds {also may be used preventively by starting a day or so before ascent}.
- ⓘ Occurs above 2000 metres. Dehydration, tobacco and alcohol must be avoided.

CHRONIC

[MONGE'S DISEASE]

⨯ Coca 30c bd.
ⓘ Occurs in residents of high places. Relocation to a lower altitude is recommended.

Mourning

See: Bereavement.

Mouth ulcers

See: Aphthous ulcers.

Mucocele

⨯ Silicea 12c bd.

Multiple sclerosis

⨯ Cannabis indica 30c tds {in general}.
⨯ Mercurius solubilis 6c bd.
Borage Oil 1g bd.
Flax Seed Oil 1g tds.
ⓘ A diet low in animal products but high in fish may be helpful.

Mumps

⨯ Jaborandi 30c 4h {in general}.
⨯ Pulsatilla 6c 4h {with orchitis}.

Murderous

See: Killers.

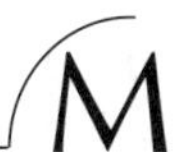

Muscae volitantes
[FLOATERS]

ⓘ Only treatment for anxiety is usually warranted.

Myalgic encephalopathy
[ME]

See: Postviral syndrome.

Myeloma, multiple

See: Cancer support; Lumbago.

Myocardial infarction

See: Collapse.

Myxoedema

See: Hypothyroidism.

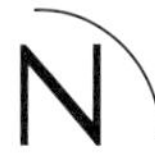

N

Nagging

- ⁂ Bach Chicory tds {possessive and selfish}.
- ⁂ Bach Beech tds {nitpicking}.
- ⁂ Bach Vine tds {dictators}.

Nail(s)

BITTEN

- ⓘ Treat as for anticipatory anxiety, chronic anxiety, or fear.

BRITTLE, COMMON

- Methyl Sulphonyl Methane [MSM/organic sulphur] 1g bd {in many cases}.
- Zinc 15mg om/bd.
- ⓘ Watch out for undiagnosed cases of hypothyroidism and iron deficiency (*see* alopecia, anaemia and Appendix 1).

CHRONIC FUNGAL INFECTIONS OF

- ❀ An oil of the following formulation is to be applied well to both the affected nails and their nail folds bd:

  Virgin Olive Oil 5ml
  Tea Tree Oil 5ml

- ⓘ Sometimes additional treatment for chronic gastrointestinal candidiasis is required (*see also* Appendix 1).

FOLD INFECTION

See: Ingrowing toenail; Paronychia.

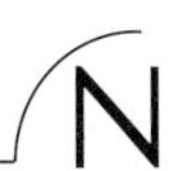

MULTIPLE WHITE SPOTS OF

[YOM KIPPUR SPOTS]

- Zinc 15mg om/bd.
- ⓘ The odd white spot may indicate simple acute trauma or an episode of acute zinc deficiency due to fasting or illness. Multiple spots are more indicative of chronic zinc deficiency, irrespective of blood levels and require the use of supplementary zinc.

YELLOW

[YELLOW NAIL SYNDROME]

- Vitamin E 400IU bd.

Narrow-mindedness

- ⁂ Bach Beech tds {critical of ideas that appear faulty}.
- ⁂ Bach Rock Water {excessive rigidity of all ideas and body}.

Nephritis, acute

See: Glomerulonephritis.

Nephrotic syndrome

- Moducare® [plant sterols 20mg + sterolins 20mg] 1 cap tds.
- Flax Seed Oil 1g tds.

Nerve trauma

MOTOR

- ⨯ Causticum 30c bd.

SENSORY

- ⨯ Hypericum 30c bd.

Nervous breakdown

See: Anxiety and depression; Bereavement; Despair.

Nettle rash

See: Urticaria.

Neuralgia

MIGRAINOUS

See: Migrainous neuralgia.

POSTHERPETIC

- Inj Vitamin B12 [hydroxocobalamin] 500μg sc/im om.
- ⚔ Kali phosphoricum 12c bd.
- ❀ Capsaicin 0.075% cream tds/qds.

TRIGEMINAL

- Inj Vitamin B12 [hydroxocobalamin] 1000μg sc/im once weekly.
- ❀ Capsaicin 0.075% cream tds/qds.

Neuritis, alcoholic

- Vitamin B complex high potency as directed.
- ⚔ Phosphorus 6c bd.
- ⓘ *See also* alcohol, alcoholism.

Neuropathy, diabetic

See: Diabetic neuropathy.

News, bad, ill effects of receiving

See: Bad news.

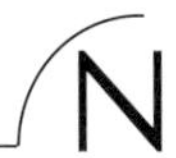

Night blindness

- Vitamin A 3000μg om.
- Zinc 15mg om/bd.
- Colladeen® [Anthocyanadin Complex] 80mg om.

Nightmares

See: Dreams.

Nipples, cracked/sore, during lactation

- ❀ Calendula officinalis 5% cream bd.
- ⨯ Castor equi 6c tds.

Nits

See: Head-lice.

Noise, sensitivity to

- ⨯ Borax 30c tds {intolerance of loud noise}.
- ⨯ Theridion 30c tds {intolerance of the slightest noise}.

Nosebleed

See: Epistaxis.

Nosiness

See: Inquisitive.

Nostalgia, unpleasant

- ✳ Bach Honeysuckle tds.

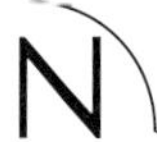

Nuisance, genuinely apologises for being a

⋇ Bach Pine tds.

Nymphomania

See: Sex.

Obesity and weight loss, adjunctive therapy in

- Chitosan 1–2g before food.
- Griffonia bean as L-5 hydroxytryptophan 50mg on {reducing to every second or third night, if diurnal drowsiness occurs}.
- Commiphora mukul [gum guggulu] as guggulsterones 25–30mg tds.
- ⓘ Exercise is always important with any therapy. Treatment for anxiety or depressive illness may be warranted in those who consistently overeat. Beware of cases of occult hypothyroidism or anorexia/bulimia nervosa presenting for treatment.

Obsessive-compulsive disorder

- Hypericum perforatum as hypericin 500μg bd.
- ⓘ *See also* hand-washing, hygiene.

Obstinacy

- Bach Beech tds {feel they know better in most things}.
- Bach Vervain tds {refuses to concede on matters of conscience}.
- Bach Vine tds {refuses advice from those perceived as lesser mortals}.

Odour of body, offensive

- Sulphur 30c bd {hot persons; may aggravate eczema}.
- Psorinum 6c bd {chilly persons}.
- ⓘ Avoiding pungent foods and good personal hygiene are essential.

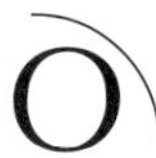

Oedema

ANGIOEDEMA

ⓘ Treat as for chronic urticaria.

CARDIAC

See: Heart failure.

FEMALE HORMONAL

See: Fluid retention.

FLIGHT

❀ Urtica dioica 1:5 Ø 5gtt tds {also preventive when taken for 24 hours prior to flight and during}.

HEAT

See: Heat oedema.

LYMPHATIC

See: Lymphoedema.

VARICOSE

See: Varicose veins.

Old links, to assist in the breaking of

⁂ Bach Walnut tds.

Opportunities, loss of

⁂ Bach Scleranthus tds {swayed between two possibilities}.
⁂ Bach Wild Oat tds {uncertain about correct path in life}.
⁂ Bach Cerato tds {lack of faith in own judgment}.

- Bach Larch tds {lack of confidence but not ability}.
- Bach Gentian tds {easily discouraged}.

Orange palms

- A sign of carrot addiction, sometimes seen in those with anorexia nervosa. It can cause serious poisoning.

Orchitis, acute

- Pulsatilla 6c 4h {in general}.
- Clematis erecta 30c 6h.

Orf

See: Ecthyma contagiosum.

Osgood–Schlatter's disease

- Calcarea phosphorica 12c om and Calcarea fluorica 12c on.
- Vitamin E 400IU om plus Selenium 50μg tds.
- Inj Ruta graveolens 200c 0.5ml sc over tibial tuberosity once weekly.

Osteitis, dental

See: Dry socket.

Osteoarthritis

- Glucosamine sulphate 1g bd {may take up to 90 days to work}.
- Chondroitin sulphate 1200mg om.
- Cod Liver Oil 1g om.
- Zingiber officinalis 1:2 Ø 10gtt tds.

- ❀ Vitex agnus-castus standardized 10:1 extract 100mg om {prevention of postmenopausal osteoarthritis of weight-bearing joints}.
- ❀ Salix alba FE 1–3ml tds prn.
- ⨯ Rhus toxicodendron 30c tds {damp-aggravated, with stiffness and pain better for light exercise}.
- ⨯ Lueticum 30c on {pains worse at night}.
- ❀ PZ cream [formula given under bunion] topically tds to superficial joints, e.g. knee.
- Inj Ruta graveolens 200c 0.25ml sc to acupoints of relevant joints {maximum 4ml} once weekly.
- ⓘ The diet should be low in meat and dairy products. Some improve by avoiding capsicums, tomatoes, aubergines (eggplants), and citrus fruits and their juices.

Osteochondrosis

See: Osgood-Schlatter's disease; Scheuermann's disease.

Osteogenesis imperfecta

- ⨯ Symphytum 6c bd.

Osteoma

- ⨯ Calcarea fluorica 12c bd.

Osteomyelitis

- ⨯ Silicea 12c bd {to promote the expulsion of sequestra}.

Osteoporosis

- Osteogard® [Calcium 500mg + Magnesium 250mg + Boron 1.5mg] 1 tab om/bd.
- Cod Liver Oil 1g om.

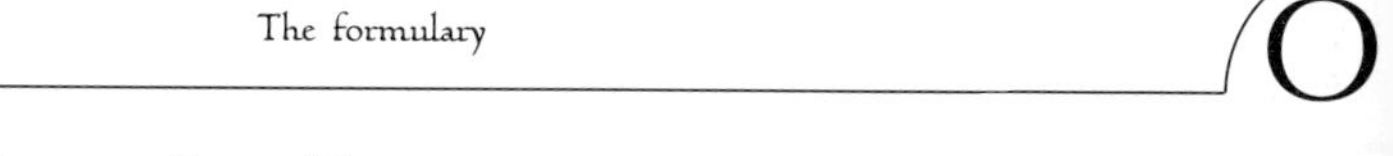

- Phytomenadione 10mg om.
- Calcarea fluorica 6c bd.
- Vitex agnus-castus standardized 10:1 extract 100mg om.
- ⓘ The above may be useful preventively as well. Less meat, more fish (especially canned) and soya products may help. Caffeine should be restricted as well as salt (except in hot climates).

Ostracized

- Bach Holly tds {due to overtly angry and hateful attitude}.
- Bach Heather tds {due to incessant talking}.
- Bach Beech tds {due to being overly critical}.
- Bach Chicory tds {due to being excessively demanding}.
- Bach Willow tds {due to persistent grumbling}.

Otitis

EXTERNA, CHRONIC

- Lavender Oil 2gtt each ear bd/tds.
- ⓘ The condition is sometimes associated with chronic gastrointestinal candidiasis, for which additional treatment is required. Otherwise, internal therapy along the lines given for eczema may be indicated.

MEDIA, ACUTE – 1ST STAGE: WITH MUCH PAIN

- Medorrhinum 200c 12h three doses only {in general; will often abort an attack}.
- Belladonna 30c 2h.
- Calcarea carbonica 30c 4h {if either of the above fails to relieve}.

MEDIA, ACUTE – 2ND STAGE: EXTERNAL DISCHARGE

- Calcarea carbonica 30c bd {in general}.
- Silicea 12c bd.

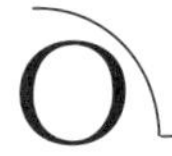

MEDIA, CHRONIC

- ⚔ Kali muriaticum 6c bd.
- ⚔ Agraphis nutans 6c bd.
- ⓘ Additional treatment along the lines given for chronic nasal catarrh of children is usually indicated.

MEDIA, PREVENTION OF RECURRENT ACUTE

- ⓘ Treatment along the lines given for chronic nasal catarrh of children is usually indicated and/or preventive therapy for common colds.

Otosclerosis

- ⚔ Calcarea fluorica 12c bd.

Ovary

CYST OF

See: Cyst.

POLYCYSTIC

See: Polycystic ovary syndrome.

Overindulgence, ill effects of

- ⚔ Nux vomica 30c 2h prn {from food in general/alcohol}.
- ⚔ Pulsatilla 30c 2h prn {from greasy or fatty foods in particular}.
- ❀ Crataegus oxycanthoides FE 5gtt tds prn {with abdominal bloating}.

Overwhelmed

- ✳ Bach Elm tds {by responsibilities/duties}.
- ✳ Bach Centaury tds {by complying with the excessive demands of others}.

- ⋇ Bach Impatiens tds {by external interference when attempting to complete a task}.
- ⋇ Bach Vervain tds {by voluntarily taking on too many jobs at once}.

Overwork

- ⋇ Bach Oak tds {from duty}.
- ⋇ Bach Vervain tds {from voluntarily taking on too many jobs at once}.
- ⋇ Bach Centaury tds {from complying with the excessive demands of others}.
- ⋇ Bach Olive tds {utter exhaustion from}.
- ⓘ *See also* common exhaustion.

P

Palsy

See: Bell's palsy; Nerve trauma; Stroke.

Pancreatitis

ACUTE

⨯ Belladonna 30c tds.

CHRONIC

⨯ Phosphorus 12c bd {in general}.
⨯ Iodum 12 c bd.
Pancreatic enzymatic supplements as directed.

Panic attack

ⓘ Treat acute attack as for fright. If recurrent, treat as for anxiety.

Paranoia

❀ Hypericum perforatum as hypericin 500μg bd.
⁕ Bach Holly tds {suspicious of the motives of others}.
⁕ Bach Cherry Plum tds {with violent tendencies}.
ⓘ *See also* paranoid schizophrenia.

Parkinson's disease

NADH [Nicotinamide Adenine Dinucleotide/Coenzyme 1] 0.14mg per kg body weight om.

Paronychia

ACUTE

[WHITLOW]

⚔ Gunpowder 6c tds.
ⓘ Drainage via the nail-fold is recommended.

CHRONIC

❀ The following formula should be applied topically bd:

Propolis 1:1 Ø	10ml
Tea Tree Oil	30gtt

⚔ Silicea 12c bd.
ⓘ The ingrowing toenail is a special variety that may warrant other treatment.

Past

✳ Bach Honeysuckle tds {dwells upon excessively}.
✳ Bach Walnut tds {to help cut ties with}.

Path in life, uncertainty about correct

✳ Bach Wild Oat tds {assists in choosing a career}.

Peace, avoidance of

✳ Bach Agrimony tds {always seeking wild distraction}.
✳ Bach Heather tds {always seeking conversation}.

Pediculosis

See: Crabs; Head-lice.

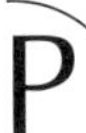

Pelvic sepsis, chronic

⚔ Tilea europoea 30c bd.

Peptic ulcer

ⓘ Treat medicinally and dietetically as for non-ulcer dyspepsia.

Perfectionism

✳ Bach Vine tds {demands all should do as they are told}.
✳ Bach Beech tds {fussy about detail}.
✳ Bach Rock Water tds {self-perfectionism}.
✳ Bach Crab Apple tds {obsessive about cleanliness}.

Pericoronitis
[WISDOM TOOTH INFECTION]

⚔ Hepar sulph. 6c tds {without trismus}.
⚔ Cheiranthus 30c tds {with trismus}.
ⓘ Hot salt mouthwashes tds are recommended. A dental surgeon must be consulted.

Periodontal disease

See: Gingivitis.

Periods, disorders of

See: Menstrual disorders.

Perspiration, excessive

See: Sweating.

Pertussis

See: Whooping cough.

Peyronie's disease

❀ Dimethyl Sulphoxide [DMSO] 25–50% gel bd {topically}.

Pharyngitis, acute

See: Sore throat.

Phlebitis

⚔ Hamamelis virginiana 6c tds.
❀ Aesculus hippocastanum 1:5 Ø tds {topically}.
ⓘ Consider treating subsequently as for varicose veins.

Phobias

❀ Hypericum perforatum as hypericin 500μg bd.
⁂ Bach Crab Apple tds {about dirt or infection}.

Pilonidal sinus and abscess

⚔ Silicea 12c bd.

Pinworms

See: Threadworms.

Pityriasis

CAPITIS

See: Dandruff.

ROSEA

⚔ Arsenicum album 12c bd.

VERSICOLOR

❀ Neem Oil cream bd {topically}.

Pleurisy

ACUTE

⚔ Bryonia 30c tds.

STITCHING CHEST PAINS FOLLOWING

⚔ Carbo animalis 30c bd.

Pneumonia, adjunctive therapy of

⚔ { Antimonium tartaricum 30c + Phosphorus 30c } 4–6h.

⚔ Bryonia 30c in 4h alternation with the above, if pleurisy occurs.

Poison ivy/oak rash

❀ Jewelweed [Impatiens capensis] soap and spray topically as directed.

Polycystic ovary syndrome

❀ Vitex agnus-castus standardized 10:1 extract 100mg om.

⚔ Folliculinum 12c bd {in general}.

⚔ Medorrhinum 200c once fortnightly.

ⓘ *See also* hirsutism.

Polymyalgia rheumatica, adjunctive therapy of

- Moducare® [plant sterols 20mg + sterolins 20mg] 1 cap tds.
- Vitamin B6 50mg tds.
- Harpagophytum procumbens 1:5 Ø 5–10ml bd.
- Treat also as for adrenal depletion in steroid reduction phase, if recrudescence of pain occurs.

Polypus

- Medorrhinum 200c one dose fortnightly.

Postnatal depression

- Griffonia Bean Extract as L-5 hydroxytryptophan 50mg on {reducing to every second or third night, if diurnal drowsiness occurs}.
- Hypericum perforatum as hypericin 500μg bd.
- Sepia 12c bd {in general}.
- Natrum muriaticum 30c bd.

Postviral syndrome

- NADH [Nicotinamide Adenine Dinucleotide/Coenzyme 1] 0.14mg per kg body weight om.
- Inj Vitamin B12 [hydroxocobalamin] 1000μg sc/im once weekly.
- Zinc 15mg om/bd.
- Panax ginseng [Ginseng] 1:5 Ø 5ml om.
- Siberian Ginseng 1500mg om.
- Panax ginseng 6c bd.
- If the original causative organism is identifiable, then the prescription of its nosode in a potency of 30–200c can be most helpful {from once per week to once per month, according to response}.
- Wheat exclusion is helpful in some cases (*see* food allergy). Watch out for occult hypothyroidism as a contributory cause in those with a family history of thyroid disorder of any variety. *See also* chronic fatigue syndrome.

Pregnancy, nutritional supplementation in

- Folic Acid 600μg om.
- Zinc 15mg om.
- Calcium in the form of canned fish with edible bones.

Premature

EJACULATION

- ❀ Hypericum perforatum as hypericin 500μg bd.
- ⁂ Bach Pine tds.

VENTRICULAR BEATS

- Coenzyme Q10 60mg tds {this prescription should not be stopped abruptly if congestive heart failure is also present}.

Premenstrual syndrome

- ❀ Vitex agnus-castus standardized 10:1 extract 100mg om.
- Magnesium 400mg om.
- Vitamin B6 50mg bd/tds.
- Vitamin E 250IU om.
- Inj Vitamin B12 [hydroxocobalamin] 1000μg sc/im a single dose monthly 7 days before menses.
- ⨯ Sepia 12c bd.

Presbycusis

- ❀ Ginkgo biloba 1:5 Ø 2gtt per 6kg body weight bd {halve the dose in those with a past history of stroke or severe hypertension}.
- Zinc 15mg bd.

Pressure, ill effects of being under

See: Overwhelmed; Overwork.

Procrastination

- ⁂ Bach Scleranthus tds {due to general indecisiveness}.
- ⁂ Bach Larch tds {due to doubt of own ability}.
- ⁂ Bach Hornbeam tds {due to fatigue}.
- ⁂ Bach Mimulus tds {due to fear of results of decision}.
- ⁂ Bach Wild Rose tds {due to general apathy}.
- ⁂ Bach Clematis tds {due to general idleness}.

Proctitis

- Moducare® [plant sterols 20mg + sterolins 20mg] 1 cap tds.

Prolapse

RECTAL

- ⨯ Podophyllum 30c bd.

UTERINE

- ⨯ Sepia 30c bd.
- ⓘ Pelvic floor exercises and yoga can be helpful.

Prostate

INFLAMMATION OF [CHRONIC PROSTATITIS]

- ❀ Serenoa serrulata 1:5 Ø 30gtt bd.
- ❀ Zea mays 1:5 Ø 30gtt bd.
- ⨯ E. coli 6c bd {in general}.
- ⨯ Lycopodium 12c bd.

HYPERTROPHY OF

- ❀ Serenoa serrulata 1:5 Ø 30–60gtt bd/tds.
- Zinc 15mg om/bd.
- Moducare® [plant sterols 20mg + sterolins 20mg] 1 cap tds.

Proving, clinical

ⓘ This term refers to new symptoms which develop during homoeopathic treatment which are characteristic of the remedy rather than the patient - a form of side-effect. It may result from over-sensitivity of the subject, or from giving the remedy in too high a potency, too frequently or for too long a period. The best initial course of action is usually to stop the remedy and wait for the symptoms to remit. Thereafter, the treatment may be recommenced in a less aggressive manner, a completely different prescription sought, or nothing further given at all.

Pruritus, idiopathic (without rash)

⚔ Caladium 30c tds {anogenital}.
⚔ Ambra grisea 30c tds {anogenital}.
ⓘ Especially in the elderly, this may be a sign of iron deficiency (*see* anaemia and Appendix 1), which must be treated accordingly.

Psoriasis

❀ Smilax spp. 1:5 Ø 30gtt bd/tds.
❀ Pycnogenol® [Pine Bark Extract] 20mg om/bd.
❀ Mahonia aquifolium 1:5 Ø bd {topically}.
❀ Aloë vera gel bd {topically}.
🌶 Flax Seed Oil 1g tds.
⚔ Arsenicum album 6c bd {with large scales}.
⚔ Arsenicum iodatum 6c bd {small non-powdery scales}.
⚔ Hydrocotyle asiatica 6c bd {circular, thick plaques with much itching}.
ⓘ In men, alcohol consumption should be restricted. Some cases seem to be associated with food allergy and gluten exclusion is worth trying for at least a month or so. Where there is a psychological base, consider also treatment of anxiety. Bathing in soft water may be beneficial.

Puberty, delayed

⨯ Pituitarin 30c om.

Pulpitis, acute/chronic dental

⨯ Hepar sulph. 200c tds {acute}/bd {chronic}.
ⓘ The tooth is sensitive to hot and cold. A dental surgeon must be consulted. *See* toothache.

Purpura, idiopathic thrombocytopenic

⨯ Phosphorus 30c bd.
🌶 Moducare® [plant sterols 20mg + sterolins 20mg] 1 cap tds.
ⓘ Arnica is ineffective in this condition.

Q

Querying/questioning

- ⁂ Bach Holly tds {from gross suspicion}.
- ⁂ Bach Willow tds {from general dissatisfaction}.
- ⁂ Bach Vine tds {from gross arrogance}.
- ⁂ Bach Beech tds {from sense of knowing better}.
- ⁂ Bach Vervain tds {from genuine interest and enthusiasm}.
- ⁂ Bach Cerato tds {repeatedly for reassurance}.

Quinsy
[PERITONSILLAR ABSCESS]

- ⨯ Lachesis 12c 2h {in general}.
- ⨯ Hepar sulph. 3c 2h three doses only {dose=4 tab adult/2 tab child}.

R

Rage, excessive

- ⁜ Bach Holly tds {from hatred or jealousy}.
- ⁜ Bach Cherry Plum tds {irrational, with violence}.
- ⁜ Bach Vervain tds {from anger over injustices to others}.
- ⁜ Bach Impatiens tds {from general irritability or impatience}.
- ⁜ Bach Vine tds {from compromise of own authority}.

Ranula

- ⨯ Thuja 6c bd.
- ⨯ Calcarea carbonica 12c bd.

Rape, psychological disorders following

- ⨯ Staphisagria 12c bd {in general}.
- ⁜ Bach Star of Bethlehem 1h prn-tds {shock}.
- ⁜ Bach Crab Apple tds {sense of uncleanliness}.
- ⁜ Bach Rock Rose tds {nightmares}.
- ⁜ Bach White Chestnut tds {preoccupied with what has happened}.
- ⁜ Bach Pine tds {guilt}.

Raynaud's disease and phenomenon

- Evening Primrose Oil 1g tds.
- Garlic Extract standardized 300–450mg bd.
- Flax Seed Oil 1g tds.
- ⨯ Silicea 12c bd {in general}.
- ⨯ Secale 6c tds.
- L-Carnitine 500mg tds.
- ⓘ In Raynaud's phenomenon, the associated condition must also be treated.

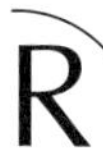

Reassurance, desires much

- ⋇ Bach Larch tds {from lack of confidence, not ability}.
- ⋇ Bach Wild Oat tds {from inability to find a correct path in life}.
- ⋇ Bach Cerato tds {from all and sundry}.
- ⋇ Bach Mimulus tds {from fear of consequences of own actions}.

Rectal prolapse

See: Prolapse.

Reflux oesophagitis

See: Hiatus hernia.

Regrets

- ⋇ Bach Honeysuckle tds {the past}.
- ⋇ Bach Pine tds {the present}.
- ⋇ Bach Walnut tds {a change of circumstances}.

Reiter's syndrome

- ⨯ Rhus toxicodendron 30c tds.

Reminisces constantly

- ⋇ Bach Honeysuckle tds.

Repetition, constant

- ⋇ Bach Cerato tds {of question, for reassurance}.
- ⋇ Bach Vervain tds {verbal, of ideas and good causes}.
- ⋇ Bach Impatiens tds {verbal, to hurry others}.
- ⋇ Bach Heather tds {self-centred verbal diarrhoea}.

※ Bach Cherry Plum tds {of previous bad decisions or mistakes}.

Repetitive strain injury
[RSI]

⨯ Ruta graveolens 30c tds.
Glucosamine sulphate 1g bd.
Inj Ruta graveolens 200c sc 0.5–1ml over most tender point(s) once weekly {maximum 4ml}.

Resentment

※ Bach Willow tds {grumbling, over most things}.
※ Bach Holly tds {from overt jealousy, or with wish of vengeance}.
※ Bach Chicory tds {when not the centre of attention}.
※ Bach Vervain tds {over injustices to others}.

Resignation

※ Bach Wild Rose tds {to dull, monotonous existence}.
※ Bach Gorse tds {to never getting well again}.

Responsibility

※ Bach Elm tds {overwhelmed by}.
※ Bach Oak tds {soldiers on, out of sense of}.
※ Bach Larch tds {although capable, avoids}.
※ Bach Vervain tds {voluntarily takes on too much}.

Restless leg syndrome

⨯ Zincum metallicum 12c bd {men}.
ⓘ In women this is often due to iron deficiency. *See* anaemia and Appendix 1.

Restraint, excessive self-

- ⋇ Bach Rock Water tds.

Retinopathy, diabetic and hypertensive

- ⓘ Treat as given under diabetic retinopathy.

Retirement

- ⋇ Bach Walnut tds {to help adaptation to}.
- ⋇ Bach Wild Oat tds {uncertainty about the future}.
- ⋇ Bach Vervain tds {cannot switch off from busy previous life}.
- ⋇ Bach Honeysuckle tds {constant reminiscence about the past}.
- ⋇ Bach Wild Rose tds {unmotivated, with resignation to boredom}.
- ⋇ Bach Holly tds {resentful of enforced}.

Revenge

- ⋇ Bach Holly tds.

Rheumatism, intercostal

See: Intercostal rheumatism.

Rheumatoid arthritis

See: Arthritis.

Rhinitis

See: Catarrh; Colds; Hay fever; Polypus; Sinusitis.

Ridicule, tendency to

- ⋇ Bach Holly tds {spitefully}.
- ⋇ Bach Beech tds {over the imperfections of others}.
- ⋇ Bach Vine tds {in an attempt to dominate}.

Ringworm

- ❀ Neem Oil cream tds.
- ❀ Tea Tree Oil 10% cream tds.
- ⨯ Bacillinum 100c once fortnightly.

Risks, excited by

- ⋇ Bach Agrimony tds {to hide inner mental turmoil}.
- ⋇ Bach Vervain tds {in the service of others}.

Rosacea

- ❀ Smilax spp. 1:5 Ø 30gtt bd/tds

Rudeness

See: Impudence.

Rut, feeling in a

- ⋇ Bach Wild Rose tds {resigned to monotonous existence}.
- ⋇ Bach Wild Oat tds {from failure to decide correct path in life}.
- ⋇ Bach Gorse tds {from resignation to illness}.
- ⋇ Bach Clematis tds {but does not care}.

Ruthlessness

- ⋇ Bach Vine tds {from a dictatorial personality}.
- ⋇ Bach Holly tds {from jealousy or hatred}.
- ⋇ Bach Cherry Plum tds {from irrational and uncontrollable violence}.

S

SAD
[SEASONAL AFFECTIVE DISORDER]

- ❀ Hypericum perforatum as hypericin 500μg bd.

Sadism

- ⨯ Staphisagria 12c bd {with sexual undertones}.
- ⁂ Bach Vine tds {from dictatorship; Joseph Stalin types}.
- ⁂ Bach Holly tds {from spite or revenge}.
- ⁂ Bach Rock Water tds {from matters of principle; religious fanatics}.

Salivary calculi

- ⨯ Calcarea fluorica 12c bd.

Sanctimony

- ⁂ Bach Rock Water tds {self-perfectionistic}.
- ⁂ Bach Vine tds {dictatorial delivery of edicts and dogma}.
- ⁂ Bach Beech tds {preaches precision}.
- ⁂ Bach Vervain tds {preaches morality and ethics}.

Sanity, fear for own

- ⁂ Bach Cherry Plum tds.

Sarcasm, excessive

- ⁂ Bach Chicory tds {to gain attention for self}.
- ⁂ Bach Vine tds {to subjugate others}.

- Bach Beech tds {about minor mistakes}.
- Bach Holly tds {from jealousy or greed}.
- Bach Willow tds {from general resentment}.

Sarcoidosis

- Bacillinum 30c once weekly.

Scabies

- Neem Oil Cream on after a bath/shower.
- Silicea 12c bd.

Scalds

See: Burns and scalds.

Scarlatina

[SCARLET FEVER]

- Belladonna 30c tds and Apis mellifica 30c on.

Scars, to reduce

- Vitamin E cream bd {topically}.
- Thiosinaminum 6c bd.

Scepticism, excessive

- Bach Gorse tds {about the ability of anyone to cure them}.
- Bach Vine tds {about any ideas contrary to their own}.
- Bach Beech tds {about the competence of others}.
- Bach Holly tds {about the good intentions of others}.

Scheuermann's disease
[SPINAL OSTEOCHONDRITIS]

- ✕ Calcarea fluorica 12c bd.
- ✐ Glucosamine sulphate 1g bd.
- ✐ Chondroitin sulphate 1200mg om.

Schistosomiasis

See: Bilharzia.

Schizophrenia, paranoid

- ❀ Hypericum perforatum as hypericin 500µg bd {may act synergistically with current medication!}
- ✐ Flax Seed Oil 1g tds.
- ⓘ Bach Flower Remedies are a useful adjunctive therapy. *See also* paranoia.

Sciatica

- ✕ Colocynthis 30c 2h prn {left-sided}.
- ✕ Magnesia phosphorica 30c 2h prn {right-sided}.
- ✕ Ammonium muriaticum 6c 2h prn {from prolonged immobility}.
- ✕ Arsenicum album 6c tds {in the elderly}.
- ⸸ Inj Ruta graveolens 200c 0.5–1ml sc to relevant acupoints {maximum 4ml} once or twice weekly.
- ✐ Glucosamine sulphate 1g bd {chronic cases}.
- ⓘ Normal acupuncture and chiropractic or osteopathic manipulation are often helpful.

Scleroderma

- ❀ Dimethyl Sulphoxide [DMSO] 25–50% gel bd {topically}.

Seasickness

See: Motion sickness.

Seasonal affective disorder

See: SAD.

Seborrhoeic dermatitis

❀ Smilax spp. 1:5 Ø 30gtt bd/tds.
❀ Aloë vera gel bd {topically}.
ⓘ There may be multiple causative factors, which require additional treatment or elimination: anxiety; chronic fatigue; topical reaction to soaps, hard water or perfumes; reaction to ingested or inhaled chemicals; chronic gastrointestinal candidiasis.

Selfishness

⁜ Bach Chicory tds {must be constant centre of attention}.
⁜ Bach Heather tds {endless gabbling about own problems}.
⁜ Bach Willow tds {only concerned with own grievances}.
⁜ Bach Vine tds {only generous to the sycophant}.

Servility

⁜ Bach Cerato tds {weak and easily imposed upon}.
⁜ Bach Pine tds {easily made to feel guilty}.
⁜ Bach Agrimony tds {easily dragged into dangerous activities or cults, to hide from inner emotional turmoil}.

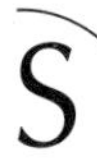

Set-backs

- ⚹ Bach Oak tds {hides exasperation and soldiers on}.
- ⚹ Bach Gentian tds {easily put off by minor}.
- ⚹ Bach Gorse tds {feels things will not right themselves}.
- ⚹ Bach Mimulus tds {feels frightened by}.

Sex

- ⨯ Staphisagria 12c {lack of, with frustration}.
- ⚹ Bach Crab Apple tds {feels dirty from}.
- ⚹ Bach Mimulus tds {afraid of consequences of}.
- ⚹ Bach Larch tds {doubts competence in}.
- ⚹ Bach Water Violet tds {dislike of sharing oneself in}.
- ⚹ Bach Wild Rose tds {too generally apathetic to be interested in}.
- ⚹ Bach Hornbeam tds {fatigue from overindulgence in}.
- ⚹ Bach Agrimony tds {seeks risky sexual activities to hide deep inner emotional turmoil}.
- ⚹ Bach Impatiens tds {too quick}.
- ⚹ Bach Vervain tds {over-excited by sexual images}.
- ⚹ Bach Vine tds {excessively dominant in}.
- ⚹ Bach Scleranthus tds {confused sexuality}.
- ⓘ *See also* sexual abuse, libido.

Shame, excessive

- ⚹ Bach Pine tds {feels unwarranted degree of guilt}.
- ⚹ Bach Crab Apple tds {feels dirty and disgusting}.

Shigellosis

See: Dysentery.

Shin splints

- ⨯ Ruta graveolens 30c tds.
- ❀ PZ cream [formula given under bunion] applied topically tds/qds.
- ⓘ Reduction of exercise is important.

Shingles
[HERPES ZOSTER]

⚔ Ranunculus bulbosus 100c tds.
Inj Vitamin B12 [hydroxocobalamin] 500μg sc/im om.
❀ If affected, the eye may be protected with eye-drops of the formula given under conjunctivitis.
ⓘ *See also* postherpetic neuralgia.

Shock

See: Collapse; Fright; Bad news.

Shoulder, frozen

⚔ Calcarea fluorica 12c bd {in general}.
⚔ Thiosinaminum 6c bd.
Glucosamine sulphate 1g bd.
Inj Ruta graveolens 200c 0.5–1ml sc to tender points around shoulder {maximum 4ml} once or twice weekly.
ⓘ Manipulation and breaking of adhesions plus chiropractic reduction of thoracic vertebral subluxations also should be considered. Normal acupuncture can be helpful.

Shows-off

✳ Bach Vine tds {to assert dominance}.
✳ Bach Vervain tds {to assert enthusiasm}.
✳ Bach Agrimony tds {to hide inner distress}.
✳ Bach Chicory tds {to gain attention}.

Sialectasis

⚔ Calcarea fluorica 12c bd.

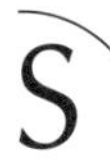

Sinus, pilonidal

See: Pilonidal sinus and abscess.

Sinusitis

ACUTE

- ⨯ { Kali iodatum 12c + Silicea 12c + Kali bichromicum 12c } tds.
- ❀ Zingiber officinalis 1:2 Ø 20gtt tds plus Echinacea angustifolia FE 20gtt tds.

CHRONIC

- ❀ Ginkgo biloba 1:5 Ø 2gtt per 6kg body weight bd {halve the dose in those with a past history of stroke or severe hypertension}.
- Coenzyme Q10 30mg om/bd/tds.
- Pantothenic Acid 250mg bd {allergic type only}.
- ⨯ Silicea 12c bd {in chilly types}.
- ⨯ House Dust Mite 30c bd {allergy to the mite}.
- ⨯ Pulsatilla 6c bd {in hot types}.
- ⨯ Medorrhinum 200c once fortnightly {sinusitis better for sea air; polyps}.
- ⓘ Cow's milk product exclusion is helpful in some cases. *See also* allergy, food allergy. Beware of chronic gastrointestinal candidiasis as a possible causative factor requiring additional treatment.

Sjögren's syndrome

- ⨯ Natrum muriaticum 12-30c bd {in general}.
- ⨯ Rhus toxicodendron 30-200c tds {with inflammatory arthritis}.

Sleep

APNOEA

See: Snoring.

GENERAL DISTURBANCES OF

See: Insomnia.

Smell and taste, idiopathic chronic loss of

- Zinc 15mg bd {full dose must be taken; may take over 12 months to work}.
- ⓘ Also treat for chronic sinusitis, if present.

Smells, excessive sensitivity to

- Nux vomica 30c tds {to smells in general}.
- Ignatia 30c tds {to tobacco smoke}.

Snobbery

- Bach Chicory tds {self-centred attention seekers}.
- Bach Rock Water tds {bigoted intellectual snobs}.
- Bach Vine tds {ruling class snobs}.
- Bach Beech tds {concerning those of lesser ability}.

Snoring

- ⓘ Many cases improve with the exclusion of cow's milk products (*see* food allergy). Also treatment may follow the lines given under chronic sinusitis.

Sore throat, common acute

- Mercurius corrosivus 30c tds {severe}.
- Phytolacca 30c tds {with sore submandibular lymph nodes}.
- ❀ Zingiber officinalis 1:2 Ø 20gtt tds plus Echinacea angustifolia FE 20gtt tds.
- ⓘ Sore throats due to glandular fever (infectious mononucleosis), quinsy and acute laryngitis are usually unresponsive to the above, and require other measures.

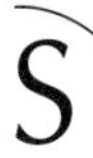

Spiteful

See: Bitchiness.

Splinters

See: Foreign bodies.

Spondylitis, ankylosing

See: Ankylosing spondylitis.

Spondylosis, cervical

ⓘ Treat as for osteoarthritis.

Sprain

ACUTE

⨯ Arnica 30c 1–4h {of any joint}.
⨯ Ledum 30c 1–4h {ankle}.
⨯ Ruta graveolens 30c 1–4h {wrist}.
❀ Arnica montana 1:10 Ø tds {topically only and not to broken skin; may also be diluted 1 in 5 with icy water for cold compress}.

CHRONIC

Glucosamine sulphate 1g bd.
Inj Ruta graveolens 200c 0.25–0.5ml sc over tender spots {maximum 2ml} once weekly.

Stage-fright

See: Anticipatory anxiety.

Stiff neck, common acute

- ⨯ Lachnantes 30c 2–4h.

Stings

See: Bites and stings of insects; Jellyfish stings.

Stones

See: Calculi; Colic.

Strain, muscular or ligamentous

- ⨯ Ruta graveolens 30c tds/qds {acute}.
- Inj Ruta graveolens 200c 0.5–1ml sc over tender spots {maximum 4ml} once weekly.
- ⓘ *See also* inguinal hernia.

Stress incontinence

- ⨯ Sepia 30c bd {in general}.
- ⨯ Causticum 30c bd.
- ⓘ Pelvic floor exercises and yoga may be helpful.

Strict, overly

- ⁂ Bach Chicory tds {from selfishness}.
- ⁂ Bach Vervain tds {about standards and morality}.
- ⁂ Bach Beech tds {about exactness}.
- ⁂ Bach Vine tds {tyrannical}.
- ⁂ Bach Rock Water tds {about self}.

Stricture

- ⨯ Thiosinaminum 6c bd.

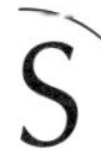

Stroke

⨯ Aconite 200c 1–4h.

Sty/stye

⨯ Pulsatilla 6c 4h {initially}.
⨯ Staphisagria 6c tds {after pain and redness are much reduced}.

Subservience

See: Servility.

Sulks

⁕ Bach Chicory tds {when not given what they want}.
⁕ Bach Willow tds {generally resentful}.

Sun

BURN

- Vitamin E cream tds prn {topically, to treat}.
- Aloë vera gel tds prn {topically, to treat}.
- Sol 30c tds {treatment}.
- Vitamin E 400IU bd plus Vitamin C 1g bd {prevention of, in addition to external anti-UV preparations}.

HEADACHE

⨯ Belladonna 30c 1–2h prn.

RASH

[SOLAR URTICARIA]

- Urtica dioica 1:5 Ø 5gtt tds {prevention}.
- Urtica urens 6c qds {treatment}.

Superiority complex

See: Aloofness.

Sweating, inappropriate

⚔ Sulphur 30c bd.

Sympathy

CRAVES

- ✳ Bach Chicory tds {spiteful if not given}.
- ✳ Bach Heather tds {garrulous demands for}.
- ✳ Bach Willow tds {but not pleased when given}.

DENIES, TO OTHERS

- ✳ Bach Vine tds {tyrannical}.
- ✳ Bach Beech tds {generally unsympathetic}.
- ✳ Bach Holly tds {out of spite or jealousy}.

Systemic and discoid lupus erythematosus, adjunctive therapy of
[SLE/DLE]

- Flax Seed Oil 2g tds.
- Moducare® [plant sterols 20mg + sterolins 20mg] 1 cap tds.
- ⓘ A vegetarian diet may be helpful, but with the avoidance of alfalfa.

T

Talkative, excessively

See: Garrulousness.

Tapeworm

❀ Cucurbita pepo [Pumpkin] seeds ground 200–400g dispersed in 1 glass of milk sweetened with honey, to be taken on an empty stomach {the patient must fast for 12 hours prior to this}. Then 2 hours later, a castor oil purge must be given in milk or fruit juice {10–20ml castor oil for adults; 5–10ml for children 5–12 years of age}. The tapeworm is usually expelled a few hours later.

Tardive dyskinesia

- Vitamin E 400IU bd.
- Manganese 15–60mg om.

Tartar

See: Calculus.

Taste, loss of

See: Smell and taste.

Teeth, sensitive [CERVICAL SENSITIVITY]

❀ Plantago major 1:5 Ø topically tds/qds prn.

ⓘ *See also* toothache.

Teething, infantile

- Chamomilla 30c 1h prn {in general}.
- Mercurius solubilis 6c tds prn {with excessive salivation}.
- Rheum 30c tds prn {with sour diarrhoea}.

Temper

IN GENERAL

See: Rage.

TANTRUMS, INFANTILE

- Chamomilla 30c tds {with desire to be carried/petted}.
- Cina 30c tds {without desire to be touched/carried/looked at}.
- ⓘ These are the main causes of breath-holding attacks in infants.

Tennis elbow

- Ruta graveolens 30c tds.
- Inj Ruta graveolens 200c 1ml sc over most tender point once weekly.
- Glucosamine sulphate 1g bd.

Tenosynovitis

- ⓘ Treat as for tennis elbow.

Terror

- Bach Rock Rose 10m prn.
- Bach Rescue Remedy 10m prn.

Testis

ACUTE INFLAMMATION OF

See: Orchitis.

UNDESCENDED

⚔ Aurum muriaticum natronatum 6c bd.

Theatrical behaviour

- ⁜ Bach Agrimony tds {to hide internal mental turmoil}.
- ⁜ Bach Holly tds {over things causing jealousy}.
- ⁜ Bach Chicory tds {to gain attention to self}.
- ⁜ Bach Vervain tds {over pet causes and injustices to others}.

Thoughts, constant and worrying

- ⁜ Bach White Chestnut tds {unable to be distracted from them}.
- ⁜ Bach Honeysuckle tds {of the past}.
- ⁜ Bach Holly tds {of jealousy or vengeance}.

Threadworms
[PINWORMS]

⚔ Cina 100c bd.

Thrombocytopenic purpura, idiopathic

See: Purpura.

Thrombosis, superficial venous

ⓘ Treat as for phlebitis.

Thrush

⨯ Borax 30–100c tds.

ⓘ Persistent or recurrent thrush usually indicates that treatment of chronic gastrointestinal candidiasis is warranted.

Thyroid disease

See: Cyst; Grave's disease; Hypothyroidism.

Time, psychological aspects of

- ⁂ Bach Clematis tds {always late through day-dreaming}.
- ⁂ Bach Wild Rose tds {always late through apathy}.
- ⁂ Bach Vervain tds {every minute must be productive}.
- ⁂ Bach Beech tds {annoyed by even the slightest delay}.
- ⁂ Bach Impatiens tds {wishes time to pass more swiftly}.
- ⁂ Bach Rock Water tds {ritualistic allocation of particular routine tasks to particular times}.

Timidity

See: Confidence.

Tinea

See: Dhobi's itch; Ringworm.

Tinnitus

- Inj Vitamin B12 [hydroxocobalamin] 1000µg sc/im once weekly {in cases produced by exposure to loud noise}.
- ❀ Ginkgo biloba 1:5 2gtt per 6kg Ø body weight bd {halve the dose in those with a past history of stroke or severe hypertension}.

- Zinc 15mg bd.
- Griffonia Bean Extract as L-5 hydroxytryptophan 50mg on {to assist sleep; reducing to every second or third night, if diurnal drowsiness occurs}.
- ⓘ Acupuncture can be helpful. Some cases improve by the treatment of any concomitant catarrh. *See also* Ménière's disease.

Toenail, ingrowing

See: Ingrowing toenail.

Tolerance, lack of

See: Intolerance.

Tongue-tied

- Bach Larch tds {from lack of confidence}.
- Bach Mimulus tds {from fear of incorrect delivery}.
- Bach Impatiens tds {from thinking ahead of talking}.
- Bach Vervain tds {from having too many things to say}.
- ⓘ *See also* anticipatory anxiety.

Tonsillar hypertrophy of children

- Baryta carbonica 12c bd {in general}.
- Silicea 12c bd {especially in catarrhal children}.
- Calcarea phosphorica 12c bd.

Tonsillitis

ACUTE

See: Sore throat.

CHRONIC

[CHRONIC CRYPTITIS]

⚔ Silicea 12c bd.

Toothache

ⓘ In prescribing for toothache, it is important to make a proper diagnosis. The most common dental causes of pain around the jaws presenting to the non-specialist are dental abscess, pulpitis, pericoronitis (wisdom tooth infection) and dry socket (post-extraction osteitis). Simple examination of the mouth will usually determine the cause. Early dental abscess without swelling and pulpitis are, however, easy to confuse, especially since the teeth are usually tender to percussion in both instances. However, *extreme sensitivity to hot or cold*, with pain persisting for many minutes/continuous pain, usually indicates that treatment should proceed along the lines given for pulpitis. Nevertheless, watch out for the odd case of trigeminal neuralgia that presents as toothache. *See also* sensitive teeth ('cervical sensitivity', where the gums have receded to expose the sensitive cementum/dentine, and though sensitive to hot/cold/brushing/sugar, the pain induced seldom lasts longer than a minute or so).

Torticollis

See: Stiff neck.

Tracheitis, acute

⚔ Causticum 12c tds {in general}.
⚔ Phosphorus 12c tds {under no circumstances should this be given in conjunction with the above}.
❀ Tussilago farfara folia as Schoenenberger Plant Juice [pyrrolizidine alkaloid-free] 10ml bd.

Travel-sickness

See: Motion sickness.

Traveller's diarrhoea

See: Diarrhoea.

Tremor, benign essential

- Flax Seed Oil 1g tds.

Trigeminal neuralgia

See: Neuralgia.

Triglycerides, high
[HYPERTRIGLYCERIDAEMIA]

- Garlic Extract standardized 300-450mg bd.
- Flax Seed Oil 1g tds.
- ❀ Commiphora mukul [gum guggulu] as guggulsterones 25-30mg tds.
- ⓘ Other ways of helping include: giving up the deadly weed, reducing alcohol consumption, combating obesity, and replacing meat with fish in the diet.

Tuberculosis

See: Lymphadenopathy.

Ugly, always feels

- ⚹ Bach Crab Apple tds.

Ulcer

See: Aphthous (Mouth); Bedsore (Decubitus); Corneal; Diabetic, peptic.

Ulcerative colitis

- ❀ Ulmus fulva/rubra powder [Slippery Elm] unadulterated, prepared and taken in the following manner:
  1. Place 2 level standard teaspoonfuls (i.e. 2 × 5 ml) in a glass jar or plastic container. Add 125ml/4 Imperial fluid ounces of cold water.
  2. Cap the jar and shake the mixture vigorously.
  3. Tip into an earthenware or glass bowl. Add 600ml/1 Imperial pint of boiling water. Stir thoroughly until the powder is dissolved. Allow to cool.
  4. Store in a covered container or bottle in the refrigerator.
  5. The dose is 1 cup/250ml tds before meals. The instructions given provide enough for 1 day. A fresh mixture should be made each morning, or, for convenience, the night before use.
- ✎ Folic Acid 5mg om {provided Vitamin B12 deficiency is absent/treated}.
- ✎ Flax Seed Oil 1g tds.
- ✎ Moducare® [plant sterols 20mg + sterolins 20mg] 1 cap tds.
- ❀ Nicotine 21mg patch 1 om {to induce remission only}.

ⓘ Cow's milk and wheat exclusion is worthy of consideration, as is a reduction of refined sugar intake, animal fat and alcohol. If the motions are loose, a reduction of fibre is indicated. Beware of cases of chronic amoebiasis misdiagnosed as ulcerative colitis.

Undescended testis

See: Testis.

Unreliability

- Bach Agrimony tds {easily persuaded to try new avenues of escape}.
- Bach Scleranthus tds {swings spontaneously from one thing to another}.
- Bach Cerato tds {seeks advice from all and sundry}.
- Bach Mimulus tds {fears the result of making a decision}.
- Bach Clematis tds {day-dreamers}.

Urethral caruncle

- Cannabis sativa 12c bd.

Urethritis, adjunctive therapy of

- Cantharis 30c tds {severe}.
- Staphisagria 30c tds.

Urinary tract infection

See: Cystitis.

Urticaria

ACUTE

- ⚔ Urtica urens 6c qds.
- ⓘ *See also* sun rash.

CHRONIC

- 💉 Inj Vitamin B12 [hydroxocobalamin] 1000μg sc/im once weekly.
- ⚔ Acidum sulphuricum 12c bd.
- ⚔ Thyroidinum 12c bd.
- ⓘ Additionally, a diet that is free of food colourants, preservatives and salicylates is a fruitful approach in some cases. Salicylates are found as flavourings in soft drinks, ice cream, chewing gum, puddings and cake mixes. They occur naturally and significantly in raisins, prunes, other dried fruits, berries, nuts and seeds. Also to be avoided are sweets containing liquorice or peppermint and certain spices and herbs - thyme, dill, oregano, turmeric (*haldi*), paprika and curry powders, including *garam masala*. Other flavourings can also bring on urticaria, such as menthol, vanilla, cinnamon and the artificial sweetener aspartame. Other possible causes, which may be occult, are dental focal sepsis and chronic gastrointestinal candidiasis, either requiring special treatment.

Uterine prolapse

See: Prolapse.

Uveitis, adjunctive therapy of

- ⚔ Mercurius corrosivus 12c tds {in general}.
- ⚔ Hepar sulph 30c tds.

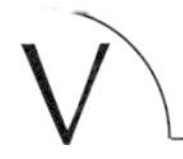

Vaccinosis, prevention of
[CHRONIC POST-IMMUNIZATION MIASM]

See: Immunization.

Vaginismus

⚔ Staphisagria 12c bd.
❋ Bach Mimulus tds {fear of pregnancy}.

Vaginitis

ATROPHIC

❀ A cream of the following formulation may be applied topically bd:

Non-lanolin base cream	50g
Propolis 1:1 Ø	40gtt

🌶 Flax Seed Oil 1g tds.
❀ Vitex agnus-castus standardized 10:1 extract 100mg om.

CANDIDA

See: Thrush.

NON-SPECIFIC

ⓘ This may be due to chronic gastrointestinal candidiasis, and appropriate treatment should be given.

TRICHOMONAS

❀ A pessary, comprising a tampon soaked in the following mixture may be inserted om/bd for 10–14 days:

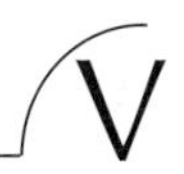

Vitamin E Oil	70ml
Tea Tree Oil	30ml

Valvular disease of heart

See: Heart.

Vanity, excessive

⁂ Bach Rock Water tds {absolutely immaculate}.
⁂ Bach Beech tds {fussy about minor details}.
⁂ Bach Chicory tds {to gain attention}.

Varicose

CELLULITES

See: Cellulitis.

ECZEMA

⨯ Sulphur 6c bd.
ⓘ And treat for varicose veins.

VEINS

- Vitamin E 250IU bd.
- Flax Seed Oil 1g tds.
- ❀ Aesculus hippocastanum 1:5 Ø tds {topically}.
- ⓘ *See also* phlebitis.

Venous

INSUFFICIENCY, CHRONIC

See: Varicose.

THROMBOSIS, SUPERFICIAL

ⓘ Treat as for phlebitis.

Verbosity

See: Garrulousness.

Verruca

❀ In the evening, after a bath, shower or footbath, the feet should be dried and the verrucae (there are usually several) abraded well with a pumice stone. Then the formula given below should be applied fairly liberally, and allowed to dry. This is best done several times, so that the verrucae acquire a lightly sun-tanned appearance. This ritual should be continued for as long as it takes for them to disappear - often up to 6 weeks, or a few months with larger ones. There is no need to scratch the solution into each verruca with a needle, and the technique is thus eminently suited to even those unfortunate cases which display many dozens of lesions on each foot:

Thuja occidentalis fluid extract	10ml
Tea Tree Oil	20 drops
Lemon Oil	20 drops

Vertigo

- ✕ Acid muriaticum 12c bd {in general}.
- ✕ Conium maculatum 30c bd.
- ✕ *See also* Ménière's disease.

Vibes, bad, over-sensitivity to

See: Bad vibes.

Vindictiveness

- ✳ Bach Holly tds {out of hatred or extreme jealousy}.
- ✳ Bach Chicory tds {when attention is turned away from self}.
- ✳ Bach Vine tds {when own authority is challenged}.

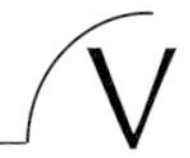

Violence

See: Rage.

Vitiligo

IDIOPATHIC

- Folic Acid 10mg om plus Vitamin B12 2000µg om.
- Folic Acid 1–10mg om plus Vitamin C 1g om by mouth, but inj Vitamin B12 [hydroxocobalamin] sc/im 1000µg fortnightly.
- L-Phenylalanine 50mg per kg body weight per day or less plus the use before exposure to sun of a 10% gel of the same.
- Khellin 120–160mg om.
- Some cases appear to depend on achlorhydria, and can improve by the administration of dilute hydrochloric acid after meals.

STEROIDAL

- Ammi visnaga D6 bd.

Voice

LOSS OF

See: Laryngitis.

TONING OF, BEFORE PERFORMANCE

- Phosphorus 30c one dose 2 hours before.

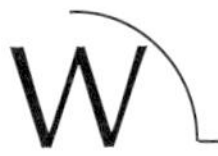

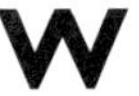

Warts

DORSAL FINGER

- ⨯ Kali carbonicum 12c bd {pale}.
- ⨯ Calcarea carbonica 12c bd {red}.
- ⨯ Medorrhinum 200c once weekly.

PALMAR OR PLANTAR

See: Verruca.

Weak-willed

See: Servility.

Wegener's granulomatosis

- ❀ Echinacea angustifolia FE 20gtt om/bd.
- ⨯ Sulphur 30c bd.

Whitlow

See: Paronychia.

Whooping cough

- ⨯ Drosera 30c tds {in general}.
- ⨯ Hydrocyanic acid 30c tds.
- ⨯ Cuprum metallicum 30c tds.

Wilson's disease

- ➶ Zinc 50mg tds.

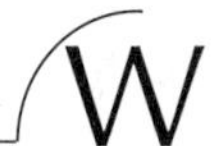

Wisdom tooth infection

See: Pericoronitis.

Workaholism

- Bach Centaury tds {from servility}.
- Bach Vervain tds {inclination to take on too much}.
- Bach Rock Water {as matter of principle}.
- Bach Oak tds {out of loyalty}.

Wound healing

LOCAL PROMOTION OF

- Calendula officinalis 5% cream bd.
- Calendula officinalis 1:5 Ø 1 in 20 as hot fomentations or irrigant om/bd.

SUPPLEMENTARY PROMOTION OF

- Zinc 15mg om/bd.
- Vitamin C 1g bd.

Wry-neck, acute

See: Stiff neck.

Xerostomia

ⓘ There are many possible causes for dry mouth, including drugs, radiotherapy and Sjögren's syndrome. Xerostomia increases the predisposition to oral thrush.

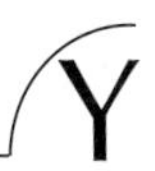

Yellow nail syndrome

See: Nail(s).

Youthfulness, obsessed with

- Bach Rock Water tds {fitness freaks}.
- Bach Agrimony tds {always seeking a wild time}.
- Bach Rock Rose tds {terror of growing old}.
- Bach Mimulus tds {fear of growing old}.
- Bach Heather tds {and with trivial ailments}.

Z

Zealotry

- Bach Rock Water tds {with utter and ruthless extremism}.
- Bach Vervain tds {with utter enthusiasm}.

Zombies

- Gelsemium 100c tds {from anticipatory anxiety; stage-fright; examination funk}.
- Bach Wild Rose tds {totally apathetic}.
- Bach Clematis tds {day-dreamers}.
- Bach Star of Bethlehem 1h prn-tds {from psychological shock}.
- Bach Hornbeam tds {from a heavy night out}.

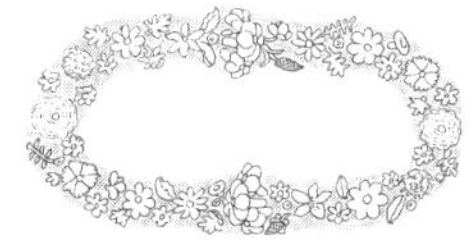

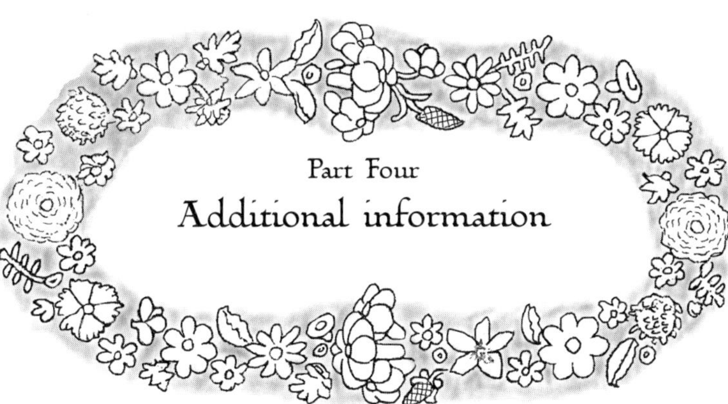

Part Four
Additional information

Appendix 1

Clinical manifestations and indications of some important syndromes

Chronic gastrointestinal candidiasis

1. Chronic fatigue.
2. Irritable bowel syndrome (abdominal bloating, excessive wind, diarrhoea, constipation).
3. Burning mouth syndrome.
4. Burning sensations anywhere.
5. Lichen planus (especially lichen planus atrophicus oris).
6. Weakness, sometimes increasing on damp days or after bathing.
7. Dizziness.
8. Headaches.
9. Irritability.
10. Depression or anxiety.
11. Diminished libido.
12. Hyperactivity in children.
13. Cold or night sweats.
14. Low-grade fever.
15. Influenza-like feeling.
16. Predisposition to upper respiratory tract infections.
17. Sore throats.
18. Recurrent or persistent thrush, cystitis or prostatitis.
19. Clear or yellow, sticky discharge from anus or vagina (vaginitis).
20. Urticarial skin lesions, not necessarily itchy.
21. Numbness and tingling of arms or legs.
22. Food allergies.

23. Alcohol aggravates symptoms.
24. Increasing allergic status in general, including hay-fever.
25. Idiosyncratic reaction to drugs, and many symptoms aggravated by antibiotics.
26. Worsening asthma.
27. Chronic sinusitis.
28. Persistent acne.
29. Persistent athlete's foot, fungal infections of nails or dhobi's itch.
30. Chronic otitis externa.
31. Hypoglycaemia and craving for sugar.
32. Joint pains and swelling.
33. Muscle pains.
34. Loss of weight.
35. Infertility, premenstrual syndrome, irregular or painful periods.
36. Associated adrenal depletion or hypothyroidism.
37. The development of the condition is, as with acute thrush, favoured by antibiotics; also by steroidal drugs of any form, and any pre-existing chronic debilitating illness or impairment of the immune system. It sometimes follows a bout of acute gastroenteritis, and may be encouraged by orthodox stomach drugs, the contraceptive pill, pregnancy and diabetes.

Fibromyalgia

Severe muscular pain

Insomnia or restless sleep	Chest pain
Fatigue	Low-grade fever
Irritable bowel syndrome	Recurrent abdominal pain
Depression	Swollen lymph nodes

Hypoglycaemia [non-diabetic/reactive]

1. Anxiety.
2. Intermittent fatigue, especially after meals.
3. Drowsiness or lack of concentration, aggravated after food.
4. Headaches, especially when hungry.
5. Excessive hunger or cravings for sugary things.
6. Sweaty palms.
7. Shakiness or tremor.
8. Depression.
9. Abdominal pain.

10. The blood sugar level is often found to be normal.
11. It is sometimes caused by chronic gastrointestinal candidiasis.

Iron deficiency

1. Heavy periods (menorrhagia).
2. A past history of iron deficiency anaemia.
3. True vegetarianism. There are plenty of bogus vegetarians around who wear the banner, but eat, as one discovers upon intensive interrogation, fish, crustaceans, bivalves or gastropods. A true vegetarian eats neither flesh nor fowl, whereas a vegan eats no animal material whatsoever, save the odd caterpillar in the lettuce; and this unwittingly so. True vegetarians and vegans are both prone to deficiencies of iron, zinc and Vitamin B12 - unless they choose not to wash their salad.
4. Pale conjunctivae or pallid tongue. Smooth de-papillated tongues come later.
5. Female alopecia.
6. *Restless leg syndrome* in females.
7. Pale nail beds.
8. Brittle nails.
9. Pale palms.
10. Generalized pruritus, especially in the elderly.
11. The blood film may be normal. The serum ferritin is always low.

Menopausal arthritis

1. Onset 38–55 years of age.
2. Symmetrical.
3. Virtually any joint may be affected below the neck, but hands are a common site.
4. Pain mild to severe.
5. Some hot swelling of joints may occur, especially hands.
6. Occasionally, some cases are sufficiently severe to resemble early rheumatoid arthritis.
7. May involve joints with established osteoarthritis.
8. Usually aggravated by hot weather and heat in general.
9. Other symptoms of the menopause may be present (e.g. infrequent periods, hot flushes).
10. Absence of rheumatoid factor (but there may be a family history of rheumatoid arthritis).

11. ESR is usually normal.
12. Blood tests may indicate menopausal changes, but the condition is sometimes premonitory of these.
13. Usually fails to respond to conventional HRT.

Reversible adrenal depletion

1. Extreme exhaustion (sometimes intermittent).
2. Poor ability to recover from relatively minor illnesses (e.g. colds).
3. Thyroid deficiency, which may be severe.
4. Dizziness or predisposition to faint; usually as a result of low blood pressure, *which fails to rise on standing*.
5. Assorted allergies, becoming more severe.
6. Diarrhoea and excessive flatulence (hence, there may be confusion with simple irritable bowel syndrome).
7. Weight loss (which may not be apparent if hypothyroidism is associated).
8. Worsening joint pain and morning stiffness (hence, there may be confusion with osteoarthritis).
9. Pallor or yellow pigmentation of the skin (due to the accumulation of carotene; a similar effect being seen in those who are addicted to carrots or carrot juice - an obsession sometimes associated with anorexia nervosa).
10. Dark rings around eyes (but not from a hangover).
11. Blood cortisol levels are usually (and unhelpfully) normal; whereas levels of DHEA [dehydroepiandrosterone] are usually low.

Appendix 2

Herb/drug/supplement interactions, side-effects and contraindications

The following table should be helpful as a quick reference to identifying possible (as opposed to probable) herb/drug/supplement interactions, documented side-effects and probable contraindications with respect to those items mentioned in The Formulary proper which are administered internally (and including possible interactive effects with certain other therapies). In fact, quite a few of the listed interactions are highly hypothetical, rather than being clinically proven. Those agents which are applied topically are not included, since the only likely reaction to them is usually one of superficial idiosyncrasy (local irritation or allergy), requiring no special consideration; only the occasional instance of systemic absorption yielding a problem. Nutritional supplements suggested in the text, which are believed at the time of writing to be essentially non-problematical, are also not included. Generally, most herbal and nutritional prescriptions derived from the text are very safe in conjunction with both drugs and each other - but there is no harm done by being cautious. Since these matters are in a continuous state of flux, you are also strongly advised either to consider adding an appropriate professional database to your computer system (e.g. IBIS, AltMed-REAX) or to consult appropriate websites (see the list at the end of this Appendix with regard to both propositions). As far as prescribing herbal preparations in pregnancy and lactation is concerned, with the few exceptions mentioned in the main text, it is best avoided by the less experienced. With regard to general anaesthesia (GA), any doubtful prescriptions should be stopped at least 3 days before the procedure, where possible.

Oral Herbal/ Nutritional Agent A	*Possible Effect on Drug/Herb/Therapy B Synergism +; Antagonism –; (notes) ↑ = increase; ↓ decrease*	*Possible Side-Effects of A or Contraindications [X] ↑ = increase; ↓ decrease*
Agropyron repens (Couchgrass)	Diuretics+ (K↓); Corticosteroids (K↓); Competitive muscle relaxants+ (if K↓); NSAIDs, Lithium (toxicity ↑)	Diuresis; [X Cardiac/Renal oedema]
Barosma betulina (Buchu)	Diuretics+ (K↓); Corticosteroids (K↓); Competitive muscle retaxants+ (if K↓); NSAIDs, Lithium (toxicity ↑); Anticoagulants+	Diuresis; GI upset
Borage Oil	Antiepileptics–	Mild GI upset; [X Gallstones]
Carduus mar. (Milk Thistle)	Drugs– (general faster detoxification of drugs in diseased liver)	
Chitosan		Diarrhoea; Fat soluble Vitamins ↓
Cinnamomum (Cinnamon)		Symptoms ↑ in chronic GI candidiasis (dose related); Allergy
Cod Liver Oil		Toxic in large amounts; [X Gallstones]
Coenzyme Q10		Not to be stopped abruptly in those with congestive heart failure
Commiphora molmol (Myrrh)	Antithyroids–; Hypoglycaemics+	Hiccup; Diarrhoea
Commiphora mukul (Guggul/Gum guggulu)	Antithyroids–; Cardiac glycosides+; Antiarrhythmics–; Antihypertensives–; Sympathomimetics+; Depolarizing muscle relaxants (risk of arrhythmias); Hypolipidaemics+	Mild GI upset; [X Liver/Inflammatory Bowel disease]
Crataegus oxycanthoides (Hawthorn berry)	Antihypertensives+; Sympathomimetics–; Cardiac glycosides+; Antiarrhythmics–; GA (BP↓); Depolarizing muscle relaxants (risk of arrhythmias); Antidiarrhoeals+	Hypotension; Nausea; Fatigue; Sweating; Hand rash; [X Hypotension]
Echinacea spp. (Purple Coneflower genus)	Immunosuppressives–	[X Multiple sclerosis, Leucoses, TB, Collagenoses, AIDS, Compositae allergy]
Evening Primrose Oil	Antiepileptics–	Mild GI upset; Headache; [X Gallstones]

Fenugreek	Hypoglycaemics+; MAOIs+; Anticoagulants+; Hypolipidaemics+; Anti-Parkinson's drugs–; Antihypertensives+; Sympathomimetics–; GA (BP↓)	
Feverfew	Anticoagulants+; Fertility treatment–	Mouth ulcers; Dry mouth; Sore tongue; Loss of/bitter taste; GI upset; Abdominal pain; Headache; Nervousness; Insomnia; Fatigue; Joint pain/stiffness; [X Compositae allergy, Pregnancy–abortifacient]
Ficorum Syrupus Compositus	Cardiac glycosides+; Antiarrhythmics–; Competitive muscle relaxants+	Colic; K↓; [X Arthritis, Urinary tract or Inflammatory Bowel disease, Intestinal obstruction]
Flax Seed Oil	Anticoagulants+	Mild GI upset; [X Gallstones]
Folic Acid	Phenytoin–	[X *Untreated* B12 deficiency]
Garlic	Anticoagulants+; Antihypertensives+; Sympathomimetics–; Hypolipidaemics+	Mild GI upset; Burning mouth syndrome
Ginkgo biloba	Anticoagulants+	Mild GI upset; Sore tongue/throat; Headache; Rosacea (dose related); Hot flushes (dose related); Intracranial haemorrhage (dose related, with PH of stroke or BP↑↑)
Ginseng, panax (Korean Ginseng)	MAOIs+; Antidepressants+/–; Tranquillizers+/–; Cardiac glycosides+; Depolarizing muscle relaxants (risk of arrhythmias); Antihypertensives+/–; Sympathomimetics+/–; Tamoxifen–; Immunosuppressives–; CNS stimulants+; Contraceptive pill–; HRT+; Anticoagulants+; GA (BP↓); Siberian Ginseng+; Hypoglycaemics+/–	Insomnia; Diarrhoea; Appetite↓; Libido↓; Mastalgia; BP↑↓; Nervousness; Postmenopausal bleeding; Amenorrhoea; Chest pain; Drug Rash; [X BP↑, Diabetes mellitus, Ca breast]
Ginseng, Siberian (Eleutherococcus)	Similar to Panax Ginseng	Similar to Panax Ginseng (but generally less aggressive in action in normal dosage)
Griffonia Bean	MAOIs+; Antidepressants+; Tranquillizers+; Hypnotics+; Hypericum+; GA+	Drowsiness; Nausea; Headache; Myalgia; Eosinophilia

continued

Oral Herbal/ Nutritional Agent A	*Possible Effect on Drug/Herb/Therapy B Synergism +; Antagonism –; (notes) ↑ = increase; ↓ decrease*	*Possible Side-Effects of A or Contraindications [X] ↑ = increase; ↓ decrease*
Gymnema sylvestre	Hypoglycaemics+	
Harpagophytum procumbens (Devil's Claw)	Cardiac glycosides+; Antiarrhythmics–; Antihypertensives+; Sympathomimetics–; Depolarizing muscle relaxants (risk of arrhythmias); Hypoglycaemics–; GA (BP↓)	Headache; Tinnitus; Anorexia; Loss of taste; Hyperglycaemia; [X Diabetes mellitus]
Hops	Tranquillizers+; Hypnotics+; GA+	[X Depressive illness]
Hypericum perforatum (St. John's Wort)	Contraceptive pill–; Antidepressants+; Griffonia Bean+; Antihypertensives+; Sympathomimetics–; Tranquillizers+; Hypnotics+; GA+	Photosensitivity
Iron (adult supp.)	Many drugs/herbs+ (if Fe↓)	Toxic to small children
L-Carnitine		[X Dialysis, Pregnancy, Lactation]
L-Lysine	(antagonized by excess Arginine in diet)	[X Pregnancy, Lactation]
Liriosma ovata (Muira Puama)	Not established	Not known
Plantago major (Greater Plantain)	Psyllium (cross allergy)	Excessive doses may cause diarrhoea and BP↑; Allergy
Plantago psyllium (Psyllium/Isphagula)	Drugs– (general delayed absorption); Plantago major (cross allergy); insulin+ (may require ↓)	Allergy; Obstruction of gut or oesophagus (in elderly, with fluid intake ↓)
Pycnogenol® (Pine Bark Extract)	Anticoagulants+	
Ruscus aculeatus (Butcher's Broom)	Diuretics+ (K↓); Corticosteroids (K↓); Competitive muscle relaxants + (if K↓); NSAIDs, Lithium (toxicity ↑)	Diuresis; Mild GI upset
Salix spp. (Willow bark)	Anticoagulants+; Methotrexate+; Acetazolomide+; Salicylates+; NSAIDs+	{≡NSAID after absorption}; Salicylate sensitivity; Drug rash; Tinnitus
Scutellaria lateriflora (Skullcap)	Antiepileptics+; Tranquillizers+; Hypnotics+; Hypolipidaemics+	Dizziness; Confusion; Seizures; Hepatotoxicity
Serenoa serrulata (Saw Palmetto berry)	Contraceptive pill–; Fertility treatment–; HRT+; Prostatic cancer therapy+; Immunosuppressives–; Tamoxifen–	Mild GI upset; [X Ca breast]
Smilax spp. (Sarsaparilla)	Anti-acne/psoriasis therapy+	Skin oil↓; Mild GI upset; Kidney irritation

Syzygium jambol.	Hypoglycaemics+	
Tinctures/FE/Ethanol	Antabuse (vomiting)	
Tussilago farfara (Coltsfoot)	Antihypertensives–; Sympathomimetics+	BP↑; Hepatotoxic and carcinogenic (with prolonged ingestion of pyrrolizidine alkaloids – which are absent in Schoenenberger Plant Juice)
Ulmus fulvus (Slippery Elm bark)		Nausea
Urtica dioica and urens (Stinging Nettle, Large/Small)	Diuretics+ (K↓); Corticosteroids (K↓); Competitive muscle relaxants + (if K↓); NSAIDs, Lithium (toxicity ↑); Hypoglycaemics+; Antihypertensives+; Sympathomimetics–; CNS depressants+; GA (BP↓)	Diuresis; Gastric irritation; Oliguria; Burning skin
Valerian	CNS depressants+; GA+	Agitation
Vitamin A		Toxic in large amounts
Vitamin B Complex		Yeast allergy (not B12)
Vitamin B12 (hydroxo-cobalamin)	(deficiency must be treated before Folic Acid given)	Headaches (injection only)
Vitamin C		Large amounts may affect kidneys
Vitamin D		Toxic in large amounts
Vitamin E	Anticoagulants+; Radiotherapy–	BP↑; Palpitations; Diarrhoea; Nausea; [X Gallstones; During radiotherapy]
Vitamin K (Phytomenadione)	Anticoagulants–	
Vitex agnus-castus (Chasteberry)	Contraceptive pill–; HRT+	Allergy; Headache; Menorrhagia
Zea mays (Cornsilk)	Diuretics+ (K↓); Corticosteroids (K↓); Competitive muscle relaxants + (if K↓); NSAIDs, Lithium (toxicity ↑); Hypoglycaemics+; Antihypertensives+; Sympathomimetics–; GA (BP↓)	Allergy; Diuresis; K↓ (with prolonged excessive use); [X K↓]
Zinc		Cramps (abdominal/limb) may occur with any dosage – prevent by giving 1mg Cu per 15mg Zn
Zingiber officinalis (Ginger root)	Cardiac glycosides+; Antiarrhythmics–; Antihypertensives+/–; Sympathomimetics+/–; GA (BP↓); Depolarizing muscle relaxants (risk of arrhythmias); Hypoglycaemics+; Anticoagulants+; Hypolipidaemics+; Anti-peptic ulcer therapy+	In large quantities may be an abortifacient (normal therapeutic doses appear to be safe)

Some relevant websites/links

http://www.pdr.net [PDR]
http://www.herbmed.org/ [herbMed]
http://www.micromedex.com/products/pd-altreaxpro.htm
[AltMed-REAX]
http://myibis.com/scripts/shopplus.cgi?DN=myibis.com&CARTID=
%cartid%&ACTION=action&FILE=/interact.html [IBIS]
http://medherb.com/ADVERSE.HTM
http://chili.rt66.com/hrbmoore/ManualsMM/HerbMedContra1.txt
http://medherb.com/DB.HTM
http://cpmcnet.columbia.edu/dept/rosenthal/Databases.html
http://www.amfoundation.org/
http://www.pitt.edu/~cbw/database.html

Appendix 3

A concise new physics of homoeopathic pharmacy

Superscript entries, e.g. 23a, refer to end-notes containing detailed technical information, and may be disregarded upon first reading. A bracketed entry in the form of (¶16) refers the reader to another numbered paragraph (in this case, paragraph 16). The details of book and web references given in the text will be found at the end of this Appendix.

Introduction

Any fruitful search for the physical nature of the homoeopathic phenomenon must be soundly based on the two founding blocks of modern physics, viz. Einsteinian relativity and quantum mechanics (Gribbin, 1999). Nevertheless, in their raw state, they do not provide us with an explanation, and thus must be modified to suit our purpose, or 'cooked', as some might unkindly say.

Einstein's General Theory of Relativity is so fundamental, that it is an inescapable ingredient of anything new that we might conjecture about the way the universe functions. However, in treating space (or space-time, more strictly) as a gravitationally warped continuum, it is difficult to apply it conceptually to the homoeopathic problem. It is necessary, therefore, to convert the continuum into an ether, or particulate structuring of space. This is actually not as straightforward as it sounds, since, amongst other things, by doing so we appear to tread on the toes of quantum mechanics. Whereas General Relativity gives us an insight into the structure of the universe on a larger scale, the moment we place it under the microscope, so to speak, we encounter the enormous inscrutability, disorganization and randomness of quantum concepts, and our particles of etheric space would seem to disappear in what has been termed 'quantum foam'. In other words, they appear not to be justifiable in terms of quantum mechanics.

Nevertheless, the truth is that, from the point of view of human conceptualization and observation, the universe is stratified. The 'outer layer' is the ordinary world which we see around us. The next 'layer' is represented by the relativistic conversion of Newtonian physics, and the one below that by quantum mechanics. Yet, as has become apparent, there is another stratum below even quantum itself.

The ordinary world layer is governed by probability or chance (as anyone who plays the lottery, or gambles otherwise, will know). In contrast, the relativistic layer is characterized by mechanistic organization, as one expects of an orderly creation of things. The quantum layer, as with the ordinary world, is again dominated by the laws of chance or probability, but in an even more exaggerated manner. Though the point is highly arguable, I have a distinct feeling that it has been placed there with some good reason, viz. to hide the truth from us of some deeper and more organized layer of a structured universe; beneath which there is, no doubt, another probabilistic layer, and beneath that another which is more organized, and so on. In fact, modern 'string theory' is an attempt to access the secrets of the layer immediately below that of quantum 'weirdness'.

Thus, when I maintain that space is particulate, I am really referring to the layer immediately below that of quantum mechanics, whilst not necessarily agreeing with all the ideas of the string theorists. In fact, it is a perfectly legitimate and traditional approach to acquire different components from several good makes of car to make one's own custom vehicle; and this is what I have effectively done. So, when I talk of the rationalization of relativity and quantum mechanics, I am referring to them as they apply to the sub-quantum layer of the conceptual universe, where its more mechanistic nature rids us of the 'fog' created by 'quantum foam'.

Unfortunately, space does not allow the full version of my theory to be printed in the present volume, and this will be published subsequently. I must, therefore, apologise for the omission of any fine details, which, in any event, are of more concern to those with a particular interest (God help them) in theoretical physics.

1. It will be reassuring to the opponents of homoeopathy that at least some of the action of its medicaments is no more than a

placebo effect; but, perhaps, more irritating for them to realise that the same applies to orthodox drugs, and to a similar degree. Although homoeopathic remedies have not been extensively tested, a limited number of properly conducted clinical trials have demonstrated that homoeopathy is capable of therapeutic effects over and above those of the simple placebo. This, coupled with the vast anecdotal evidence in its favour, and especially that emanating from veterinary circles, would suggest that we are dealing with a real, albeit mysterious, physical phenomenon. Furthermore, this phenomenon itself has two components; the first of which is the nature of the remedy, and the second, its mode of action on the living organism. Indeed, we cannot begin to explain the latter without attempting to understand the former.

2. A homoeopathic pharmaceutical system may be defined as one that largely relies on the innate memory of the water molecule for substances with which it has been in intimate contact, or for patterns imposed upon it by other means. For convenience, I shall call any source of such pharmacological information 'the donor', with water being 'the recipient'. In classical homoeopathic pharmacy, the donor is usually a solute. However, it may also be an insoluble substance repeatedly ground with lactose; the water molecules intimately bound with this molecule, plus those freely and inevitably present, acting as recipients[2a]. Nevertheless, it is also possible to prepare remedies of comparable therapeutic action in various electromagnetic devices. Here, the donor is remote from the recipient water, but information is transferred to it along wires of high conductivity. The donor may be any substance, but, rather surprisingly, can also be a pattern drawn upon a card immersed in a magnetic field, or even a series of variable resistors (potentiometers) in an electrical circuit. As bizarre as all this may seem, any proper physical theory must embrace all aspects of homoeopathic pharmaceutical technique, not merely the classical. Brief mention shall also be made with respect to the spagyric pharmaceutical technique, which has a physical basis in common with that of homoeopathy, and from which the latter undoubtedly evolved. It is also worthy of note that the preparation of Bach Flower Remedies is essentially spagyric in character.
3. Samuel Hahnemann, of course, developed his methods of preparation entirely by means of intuitive genius, not having the remotest idea of the physics involved. Indeed, it is the apparent lack of a rational basis for the therapeutic effect of

the infinitesimal that has caused many to declare it to be no more than a *reductio ad absurdum*. Nevertheless, it is unacceptable to deny the reality of something just because we are incapable of comprehending it in terms of our own limited perceptions of the universe. In fact, there have been many attempts to explain the nature of a homoeopathic remedy, and, in 1994, I produced *The Infinitesimal Dose* (Lessell, 1994) – an in-depth analysis of the various hypotheses which had been propounded over the years, together with one of my own. The latter was based in part upon various experimental investigations, spectroscopy in particular, carried out by a number of observers. Unfortunately, it would now appear that the replication of some of these has been thwarted with difficulty, with the notable exception of dielectric measurements. Since either the spectroscopic results were flawed, or, at the best, only gave the investigators but a fragmentary glimpse of a deeper physical state, I must now retract some of my original conclusions. However, I feel that the hypothesis I have subsequently developed is, hopefully, more persuasive; and, beyond that, broader in its application. For, whereas the original claimed to explain classical homoeopathic pharmacy, it failed to embrace the newer electromagnetic varieties of potentization, or even the method of sunlight energization used in the preparation of Bach Flower Remedies.

4. The minimal basic requirements for homoeopathic pharmaceutical preparation may be summarized as follows:
   A. Gravitation.
   B. A donor – which may be a substance or an electromagnetic pattern.
   C. A recipient of pharmacological information, viz. water.
   D. Immersion of the preparatory vessel in a fixed magnetic field – which may be that of the Earth itself, or supplied by a magnet or a steady electrical current.
   E. The supply of electromagnetic energy – by way of succussion, trituration, boiling, solar radiation, electricity, or from ambient electromagnetic waves or static electricity.
   F. A preparatory vessel composed of any hard material, other than iron or plain steel.
   G. A preparatory vessel which is cylindrical, paraboloid, or with a flat oval section (e.g. vial, jar, bottle, bowl, mortar, retort).
5. Before expanding these various points, it is necessary to consider some fundamental aspects of modern physics. The first of these is the matter of *hyperspace*. It is now generally

accepted that the universe has many more dimensions than just the three with which we are familiar (Gribbin, 1999). Thus, we may say that hyperspace is the sum of supra-dimensional and tri-dimensional space. So, whilst we seek the memory of the water molecule in our own space, it hides, in fact, largely where we cannot see it, viz. in the supra-dimensions. Nevertheless, we know it is there because of its biological effects. Although various attempts have been made to fathom out which part of the molecule is responsible for its memory, the truth is that it is the conformation of the water molecule taken as a whole wherein such memory resides, and then only in its occult supra-dimensional aspect. Since, however, all the dimensions of the hyperspace of water are intimately linked, it would be surprising to find no traces of this memory in our tri-dimensional world. In fact, electrical changes seem to occur, as demonstrated by dielectric measurements (Lessell, 1994: Element XI).

6. Intimately connected with the idea of space (or hyperspace) is that of *gravitation*. In accordance with Einstein's General Theory of Relativity, space curves or flexes in proximity to bodies of matter. The flexure of space, however, only reveals itself to our senses in the form of either gravity or the distortion of images; such distortion occurring due to the passage of light in a curve around a large body. In Einsteinian terms, gravity is essentially a curvature of space. In Quantum Theory, however, gravity is executed by particles called *gravitons*. Nevertheless, it would seem that gravitons are not easily found. It may be surprising for the reader to learn that we cannot understand what a remedy is before considering these matters in more detail. So, let us return to hyperspace.
7. One of the notions which logically follows from the General Theory is that 'empty' space ('space–time', technically) has some form of structure, albeit variable according to the distribution of mass and energy within it. It is, of course, very difficult to think of something with a structure that is composed of nothing. Far more probable is that primary space (see below) is composed of minute particles of mass zero which largely occupy the supra-dimensions of hyperspace, with what would be their more apparent conventional tri-dimensional manifestation seeming empty until electromagnetic waves pass through it[7a].
8. In continuity with this concept is the idea that there are, in reality, two different types of hyperspace. Firstly, there is *primary space*, which acts as the carrier of electromagnetic

energy. However, when such energy condenses to form matter, *primary space* itself is compressed to form *material space* – the second type of hyperspace. This is the space occupied by the nuclear components[8a] of atoms, and also by their dynamic electron clouds. As material space is formed, so the primary space surrounding it forms a halo of sympathetic contraction. In fact, if we were to conceptualize the particles of space as minute rubber balls, they would appear to be squeezed to a smaller size, as though in the grip of a hand; but vastly more so with respect to material space. The halo of contracted primary space does not only occur when mass is formed from energy, but also when any mass moves into a new area of hyperspace[8b].

9. This contraction of material and primary space results in a number of other physical phenomena. On the larger scale, where two celestial bodies show gravitational attraction, this is no more than the passage of attractive gravitons through supra-dimensional space between two areas of spatial contraction[9a]. This expression of *gravity*, quite naturally, also occurs when an apple falls on someone's head. In fact, even within the structure of the atom, gravitation is mediated by the same particles. With a large cosmic body, the halo of contracted primary space will reveal itself by the bending of light waves.
10. Atoms, molecules, or ions (the coarser fundamental components of matter) are thus always associated with a compression or distortion of primary space in their immediate vicinity[8a]. This distortion forms a sort of cast of the atom, molecule or ion, rather like that used by artists to encase a wax model in preparation for the pouring of bronze. This cast is, indeed, the negative spatial image of the nuclear and electronic structure. With a mixture of different molecules or ions, as occurs in herbal tinctures, the overall distortion of primary space will be an 'averaging' of the individual distortions caused by the various components (impurities and other minor solutes will have a minimal effect)[10a,b,c]. In electromagnetic potentizers, the pattern printed or drawn upon a card (which is many molecules in depth) or the setting of the resistor dials in a particular combination also results in unique distortions of primary space[10d].
11. Provided the compressed primary space is subjected to the influence of a fixed (background) magnetic field, the provision of electromagnetic energy results in the production of particles characteristic of its geometric distortion. These particles may then be stored in the supra-dimensions of the recipient (water) under appropriate conditions[11a].

12. The fixed magnetic field may be provided by that of the Earth, which is common to all methods of homoeopathic preparation, and, indeed, to those of spagyric pharmacy. In electromagnetic devices, however, either a fixed magnet or the passage of electricity is also used to supply the magnetic field, which, by its very nature, will be stronger than that supplied by the Earth, and will dwarf its contribution to the overall effect.
13. The provision of electromagnetic energy may be achieved in the following ways:
    A. Directly from the sun [Bach method; spagyric solar energization].
    B. By the agitation of polar molecules or ions during succussion, trituration or boiling[13a] [classical trituration or succussion; mechanical Korsakovian and Skinnerian devices; Bach boiling method; spagyric distillation].
    C. By the passage of electric current [active electromagnetic devices].
    D. By the utilization of ambient electromagnetic waves, such as radio-waves, or static electricity [passive/non-electrical electromagnetic devices].
14. The material composition of the preparatory vessel must be such that it does not magnetically interfere with potentization (¶16) or produce rust. It may be composed of an electrical insulator (e.g. glass, ceramic, plastic) or of any common industrial metal which is not strongly ferromagnetic (e.g. copper, bell-metal, brass, bronze, stainless steel).
15. The final basic requirement for a homoeopathic pharmaceutical system is the shape of the vessel of preparation. If this were of no relevance, we might anticipate that remedies would be commonly produced in Nature[15a,b]. Yet, this does not seem to be the case. In fact, the transfer of pharmacological information is largely restricted to a narrow band of water molecules which adhere (partially by electrical attraction) to the inner surface of the vessel. A circular section about the main axis would seem to be not only necessary for this to occur, but also one which would interfere the least.
16. The memory of water does have its limits. Fortunately for us, it neither remembers by whom it was passed nor under which circumstances. Beyond that, it cannot be imprinted with the 'casts' of lactose, alcohol or water itself[16a,b]; for, if it were able to do so, its memory would be occupied by information concerning the diluent alone, the molecules of which dominate at all stages of preparation other than that of medica-

tion onto sucrose. Although it is convenient to talk of an atomic or molecular 'cast' being transferred to water-memory, it is actually stored in a special field of supra-dimensional space in an encoded form, rather as we might store information on a magnetic tape[16c,d].

17. With regard to classical preparation in the liquid phase, the diluent is actually alcohol–water. Because of its method of production and storage (which comply with those basically required of a homoeopathic pharmaceutical system), it would seem likely that it must contain some 'old memories'. Indeed, this unwanted occupancy of water-memory must be formatted out or overwritten as part of the process of potentization. Hence, in the first stage of potentization, the delivery of electromagnetic energy via succussion results in two phenomena. Firstly, the obliteration of previous and unwanted information; and secondly, the registration of the donor molecules upon the memory of the recipient. In order for this to occur, the donor molecules must be present in large numbers along the inner surface of the potentizing vessel for them to command a place in the memory system in preference to old imprints. One of the main roles of alcohol in the process, apart from that of a preservative, would seem to be the facilitation of succussion by reducing surface tension[22a].
18. However, after a number of episodes of succussion (possibly 10 in centesimal preparations), this process comes to an abrupt halt; for, the increased level of 'electrification' of the system by the movement of polar and ionic charges causes neither formatting nor imprinting to proceed any further[13a]. If we had the patience to leave the vial in a static state for many days (or perhaps months), this would diminish and allow us to re-succuss to further advantage. On the other hand, it is far more expedient to discard most of the contents of the vial and replace them with fresh alcohol–water of lower electrical status.
19. The rationale behind serial dilution is thus twofold. Firstly, it progressively reduces the concentration of the original substance, which, in many cases, is toxic. Secondly, it allows its imprint upon the recipient to occur anew with each phase of serial succussion. In view of the latter, serial dilution might be better termed 'serial refreshment'.
20. It will be quite obvious from what has been said that the bulk of the contents of the vial is no more than a medium for generating electromagnetic energy. The really important atoms, molecules or ions of either donor or recipient are those that lie

in proximity to the vessel wall. Although the adhesion of donor molecules or ions encourages them to remain there for longer than might be expected from calculations simply based upon Avogadro's constant, they will, nevertheless, eventually succumb to repeated dilution. Even so, it would seem that the process of potentization may effectively continue for up to 100,000 times on the centesimal scale (potency CM). This can only occur by the intensification of donor information beyond the point of physical absence of originating atoms, molecules or ions. In this respect, it is apparent that water molecules already primed with such imagery continue to act as a ghostly substitute for the missing donor. Not only does the donor imprint intensify, it is also transmitted (by particles and/or non-local association) between water molecules adjacent to the inside of the vessel wall, and thus becomes equally distributed on the periphery of the liquid potency. Although some will become detached and enter the body of the diluent, at all stages of potentization, those water molecules which are potentized are always considerably outnumbered by those which are not. Even in the very earliest stages of potentization, where there are many molecules of original substance still present, the transmission of donor imprint between water molecules coexists with its direct transfer from those of the latter.

21. Whereas it might be thought that a donor image in the supra-dimensions of the water molecule might be conceptualized as a modulated wave, and its potency as a reflection of frequency, the reality is probably quite different. It is better to conceptualize a donor image as an encoded shape, initially blurred by the presence of other shapes, and which intensifies or clarifies as the latter are discarded by formatting or overwriting. This is rather like first of all holding the page of a newspaper in front of a light and trying to read it. The back of the page will show through and make the printing unclear. Then, removing the back-lighting, all becomes readable. Using broadcast sound as an analogy, the closest equivalent to donor image would be a piece of *music*; to potency, would be its *volume*; whilst the unwanted information might be thought of as *background noise*[21a].
22. In classical serial trituration and dilution with lactose[22a,b], exactly the same principles apply as for the liquid phase. Here, the all-important molecules etc. again are those closest to the internal surface of the vessel, viz. the mortar. The electrical principles involved, and the requirement for 'serial refreshment' are also similar.

23. In electromagnetic devices, neither serial succussion nor serial dilution is required. The output from the donor circuit or pattern is controlled in its flow to the recipient by means of a regulatory variable resistor (potentiometer). The obstructive electrical state which develops in the classical systems with repeated succussion does not occur here, and any potency is achievable by merely adjusting the degree of resistance offered to the passage of information. This overwrites any previously stored information (¶17), rather as one records over a used magnetic tape, but the clarity of the 'recording' (i.e. potency) is determined by the setting of the variable resistor.
24. The reason why the liquid phase of the LM scale can tolerate such a large number of effective succussions (100) at each stage is that the serial dilution factor is 1 in 50,000. The degree of 'refreshment' is thus 500 times greater than that of centesimal preparations. The development of potency (the intensity or clarity of the donor image) is greater at each stage because of this ability to supply greater amounts of energy before new diluent is required. Other differences between LM and centesimal remedies are mainly the result of differences in the mode of processing of original substances.
25. Conversely, the decimal scale is weaker in the development of potency than either the centesimal or the LM, since the degree of 'refreshment' is 10 and 5,000 times lower, respectively.
26. When purchasing remedies for professional purposes, it is important to know how they have been prepared[26a]. The type of succussion, and indeed the number of times it has been carried out at each dilution, will influence their potency. There are some remedies on the market which have been gently successed by a pendular motion of their container. These will always be weaker in effect than those more vigorously prepared. Moreover, Hahnemann recommended two vigorous succussions per centesimal dilution, whilst others recommend 10. I have no reason to doubt that two deliver close to the maximum possible effect, but suspect that a few more would do no harm. Furthermore, in order to preserve the strength of liquid potencies, it is important that they are re-energized by agitation at least once per month. However, once they have been committed to the care of sucrose, no further energization is possible by this means, as is also the case with lactose triturations.
27. Both animals and plants, as with everything else in the universe, are hyperspatial. In the tri-dimensions, such life forms exhibit a complex and dynamic electromagnetic field, which, by the very nature of things, comes to be represented

in the supra-dimensions of the organism. This supra-dimensional or 'aural' field can be partially revealed and recorded by means of Kirlian photography. This field is not only dependent on the electromagnetic activity of the body, but can also be used to regulate it[27a]. In turn, adjustments of the physical electromagnetic field lead to changes in the physical body, including the brain. The action of potentized water, the memory of which is essentially supra-dimensional, is directly upon the occult aural field, and so only indirectly upon physical processes.

28. When the body is diseased, this is reflected by changes of gestalt in the aural field. Nevertheless, when an effective therapeutic pattern is introduced, it is not the opposite of that of the disease, and the field is, thus, not directly normalized. The introduced pattern, via the material electromagnetic field, influences the physiology in its own right, to induce reversal of the pathological process; and this, in turn, leads to normalization (again via electromagnetism) of the aural field. Otherwise, as we shall see, the principle of 'like cures like' defies explanation.
29. Let us exemplify with the toxic action of mercury and its isopathic reversal. When mercury poisons the body, characteristic changes of physiology (and thus electromagnetism) occur, which then induce individual patterns to appear in the aural field. These patterns have nothing to do with the primary spatial distortion associated with mercury – they are entirely reflective of physiological disturbance, and not the more esoteric properties of the toxin. So, introducing the 'cast' of mercury, viz. homoeopathic Mercurius, into the aural field, will do nothing to normalize them directly. What actually must happen (for 'like cures like' to be valid) is that the introduced 'cast' must cause opposite effects to occur at the receptor sites of mercury. In other words, whilst atomic mercury may instruct in one way, so infinitesimal mercury instructs in exactly the opposite manner[30a].
30. Isopathy aside, material arsenic induces the production of diarrhoea, whilst homoeopathic Arsenicum can induce the cessation of certain types of the same, though not caused by this poison. Yet, when we have a case of common food poisoning, it is not cured by Arsenicum because it has the opposite pattern to that of the aural disturbance, but rather that it instructs the body in the opposite manner to material arsenic. As for the physical end of the mechanism, it is fundamentally electromagnetic[30a,b], and may be likened to wave

cancellation. Indeed, various modern electronic devices have been produced which claim to do something rather similar.

31. Perhaps more confusing are experimental or clinical 'provings' of infinitesimal remedies. Here, the infinitesimal acts as though it were the material. Thus, homoeopathic Arsenicum may unexpectedly produce diarrhoea. This is due to the 'cast' producing a 'cast' of itself in the aural field. Upon the analogy of sound, this is caused by too much 'volume' being applied, which causes distortion of that field. In very sensitive subjects, who can sometimes 'prove' any remedy, even low volume (low potency) can produce this effect. Sometimes, however, it is a summational effect induced by giving a particular remedy regularly over a long period of time, with the volume gradually building up to a critical level.
32. The usual method of administration of remedies is by mouth. Indeed, the aural manifestation of the oral (if you will excuse the pun) is a highly sensitive zone for the reception of the supra-dimensional components of the remedy. This zone also extends to the occult manifestations of the nose and pharynx.
33. Nevertheless, infinitesimal remedies may be introduced by any route, or, indeed, may be applied to the surface of the body. They may even be injected. Although a remedy is apparently capable of local action, this, by its very nature, cannot be direct. It must indirectly follow from its impression upon that part of the aural field related to the particular anatomical site of treatment or to wherever the potentized water molecules might track.
34. Rather strangely, there are some remedies which routinely act in the same manner, whether they be administered in the material or the infinitesimal. Arnica, for bruising, is one notable example, with Euphrasia for conjunctivitis being another. Both remedies exhibit similar properties when administered either topically as a lotion or internally in homoeopathic potency. This is a function of their patterning, where one half of the 'cast' is the more or less exact opposite of the other. Such ambivalence is, however, rare.
35. The antidotal effects of coffee, though by no means universal, are due to the production of a characteristic disturbance of the brain, then the electromagnetic field, and finally the aural. The distortion of the latter tends to destroy any introduced therapeutic pattern, but especially with regards to certain remedies. The 'casts' of Rhus toxicodendron and Pulsatilla are particularly susceptible. Reported antidotal problems with perfumes, peppermint and camphor probably have a similar basis.

36. The fact that suckling infants may be treated via the mother would seem to suggest that the breast-milk contains the remedy. This, however, is probably not the case. It is rather that the infant, at the time of feeding, comes under the influence of the aural field of the mother and the patterns contained therein, for which intimate contact is required.
37. In that information concerning remedies appears to be stored in a form of magnetic field in the supra-dimensions of the recipient molecule (¶16), it thus becomes transmissible via carrier electromagnetic waves[16c]. This supports the view that remedial information may be transferred via optical fibre systems to a biological system or recipient vial (Benveniste, 2001).

End-notes

[2a] Additionally, it will be shown how lactose itself (and alcohol) can also function as a recipient of donor molecular information[22a].

[7a] Einstein himself is worth quoting on this point. In an essay of 1920, entitled *Ether and Relativity*, he states: "More careful reflection teaches us that the special theory of relativity does not compel us to deny ether. We may assume the existence of an ether; only we must give up ascribing a definite state of motion to it". In other words, a particulate ether whose movements are totally random and thus unpredictable is compatible with at least Special Relativity (and, by inference, General Relativity).

[8a] The phrase 'atomic nuclear components' includes such things as protons and neutrons, their formative quarks, and the even more fundamental 'strings' (the smallest theoretical components of matter). Even between these there must exist a certain amount of primary space, which thus even pervades the nucleus itself.

[8b] This is not a fixed-lattice space, but a relativistic one. The particles of which it is composed are in a constant state of motion, as in a gas (albeit it rather slowly compared with the speed of light); and thus no individual particle can serve as a point of reference in analysing the geometry of the system (of necessity, their fundamental nature must be also to move randomly between material and primary space, and continually to exchange roles in their expression of gravitation). Furthermore, as to the question of what lies between these individual spatial particles, the answer is 'nothing' - neither material nor space - just 'void'.

[9a] The idea is that gravitation is primarily an attractive communication between different areas of compressed space, which then secondarily influences matter itself (via particles which we might term 'antigravitons'; essentially repulsive by nature, they attempt to push matter out of one zone of spatial compression into another). Concerning the mutual interaction of space and matter, the distinguished physicist John Wheeler has said "mass grips space by telling it how to curve, space grips mass by telling it how to move". When two bodies are drawn together by gravitation (such as an apple falling to the earth), it is, in a sense, their compressed spaces which are fundamentally attracted, rather than the matter of which they are composed (indeed, as I have suggested, the pull of such bodies from the material viewpoint is via repulsive forces).

[10a] This concept has significance only when it applies to those cohesive and adherent molecules which lie in close proximity to the inner surface of the preparatory vessel. Elsewhere, the molecular conformation is too subject to fragmentation and relative movement (by succussion, trituration or boiling, or even plain shaking) to be relevant[10d]. A 'collective or group cast' is composed of chaotic (meaningless/unintelligible) primary space interspersed with zones which are patterned (meaningful/intelligible)[10b]. Chaotic space results from the presence of conflicting patterns of compression from different types of molecules, and is thus characteristic of mixed solutions (in chaotic space, there is a random distribution of spatial particles with varying degrees of contraction; in a patterned space, however, grouping occurs, so that zones or layers are formed by particles in a similar state of contraction; whatever the case, the mean gravitational effect is the same for a given mass of any solute). Patterning is also a function of the geometry of the preparatory vessel, which must be cylindrical, paraboloid or flat oval. In fact, we might postulate that, in the Bach boiling method (cooling phase[10b]) or the early stages of homoeopathic centesimal or decimal liquid potentization (and trituration similarly), for any single molecular or single ionic solute Δ, $\Lambda=\Psi^n$; where Λ is its *geometric influence*, i.e. the degree of influence of Δ upon the generation of geometry or pattern from chaotic primary space within a particular 'group cast'; Ψ is its *relative concentration*={wt. per unit vol. concentration of Δ/wt. per unit vol. concentration of *all* solutes *except for* certain substances discussed later[16a,16b]}; and n is >1, and henceforth taken to be 2 (hence, $\Lambda=\Psi^2$). The *absolute*, as opposed to the relative, concentration of Δ influences the intensity (degree of spatial compression) of the patterning, rather than its geometry. Furthermore, the *relative molar concentration* may be ignored, since we are essentially concerned with gravitational effects, as determined by relative *mass* rather than relative numbers present. The *maximum* value for Λ is 1 (=100 Λ%), which can only be held by a hypothetical *single* unopposed non-ionized molecular solute M of any concentration (Ψ=1), but for very small values of *absolute* concentration, where the intensity is so low that the pattern becomes 'indecipherable'. This maximum value for Λ essentially means that the entirety of the 'cast' bears the pattern of M, and that chaotic zones are absent. The value of Λ where Ψ=0.5 (50%) is 0.25 (25 Λ%), and where Ψ=0.1 (10%) the value becomes 0.01 (1 Λ%). Since Λ-effects *summate*, it follows that, in the case of a hypothetical bimolecular solution, where both molecules are equally represented in terms of mass (Ψ=0.5), 50% of the 'cast' is patterned and 50% is chaotic. Upon the basis of the simple equation $\Lambda=\Psi^2$, the influence of impurities might be assessed and found to be considerably less than that which would be expected from linear proportional calculation. Furthermore, the greater the number of different solutes, and the more equal their concentration in terms of wt/unit vol, the greater the tendency of the 'group cast' to be chaotic (meaningless) rather than patterned (meaningful). In the case of a hypothetical solution of 10 different molecular or ionic types, where all are equally represented in terms of mass (Ψ=0.1), 10% of the 'cast' is patterned and 90% is chaotic. If we were able to process equal amounts by weight of all the soluble and recordable (¶16) molecules and ions in the world in a single vial, the result would be to produce a 'cast' comprised of virtually 100% chaotic primary space, from which no remedy could be derived. It follows that, in the potentization of herbal substances, the patterning of primary space is largely determined by the major chemical components, and only minimally by the lesser ingredients and contaminants in the diluent. The contribution of such contaminants is efficiently suppressed by using *tinctures* with a high *absolute* concentration of their major ingredients; but correct *standardization* can only

be achieved by also ensuring that the *relative* concentration of these is of some uniformity.

[10b] In the case of the Bach boiling method, no such 'group cast' is formed until the extractive boiling ceases[10c,13a]. Other than that, the random thermal vibration of molecules is largely irrelevant to the inherent geometry of the 'cast', rather as a tree is topologically the same, and recognizably so, whether swaying in the wind or static (the same might be said of the complex vibrational motion associated with the dynamics of chemical bonds (Lessell, 1994: Element VIII)). Nevertheless, we might predict that the higher the temperature, the more disorganized does the 'group cast' become and, hence, that normal potentization is best carried out in a cool environment.

[10c] In fact, boiling is a very efficient way of removing any traces of a homoeopathic remedy from a vial. This violent agitation of water molecules destroys any functional information contained in its memory (¶11) by rendering it chaotic[22a]. In fact, heating to 70°C for 30 minutes appears to achieve the same (Dana Ullman, 1995: see Benveniste). The functions of boiling in the Bach method are to secure extraction and dissolution of the chemicals contained in the plant, and the erasure of 'old memories' (¶17).

[10d] In electromagnetic potentization, geometrical information from cards or resistors, having first expressed itself by the compression of space, is then transmitted in the higher dimensions of the magnetic flow to the recipient. In that type of electromagnetic potentization where herbs, minerals, tinctures, etc. are the source of patterning, information is similarly transferred from any donor substance contained in the 'in-pot' to a recipient in an 'out-pot'. The 'rules' governing the transfer of information from such substances are as given for classical potentization[10a,16a,b]. Where the recipient is in the form of a sugar impregnated with alcohol-water, the system is essentially static, and potentization of the entire contents of the recipient vial will occur. No recordable impression of the molecules which comprise either the 'in-vial' or 'out-vial' is made, since the circularity of these vessels ensures that they are registered merely as an overall shape, rather than as a molecular 'cast'.

[11a] Although all the components of hyperspace are connected, the space in which such information is stored is different from that of the 'cast' (¶10), having its own unique set of dimensions. Speaking generally, that part of this space related to any particular molecule is occupied by imagery concerning that particular molecule alone; but, in the case of water, the space can be occupied by the imagery of other molecules[22a]. Though the 'implantation' of imagery is spontaneous/automatic in the case of most molecules, with regard to water, this can only be achieved artificially (usually pharmaceutically). As a 'cast' is a negative representation of a molecule, so the imagery contained in this space is also negative.

[13a] These techniques convert mechanical into electromagnetic energy. This involves the enforced juxtaposition of ions or the poles of polar molecules which normally would be repelled by virtue of having the same direction of polarity, positive or negative. Essentially, they are briefly forced into proximity, with consequent 'compression' of the repulsive magnetic field between them, only to be then sheared away from each other with great rapidity. The compression-shearing action on this field leads to the generation of electromagnetic particles $\acute{\varepsilon}$ which are largely supra-dimensional in character and which can be stored in the supra-dimensions of the solution/powder. This energy is somewhat akin to electricity, of which it may be conceptualized as a peculiar form. Electricity, of

course, is electronic and largely 'visible' (tri-dimensional), whereas $\acute{\varepsilon}$ is non-electronic and mainly 'invisible' (supra-dimensional). These particles should not be confused with those which convey information concerning donor image (¶11, ¶20). Whilst a proportion of $\acute{\varepsilon}$ is utilized in the production of the latter, the surplus is largely stored, with the preparatory vessel and its contents acting as a type of capacitor. As suggested elsewhere, this in itself can lead to some interesting problems (¶18). Unlike electricity, $\acute{\varepsilon}$ particles are not subject to earthing in a metallic vessel, and their retention may be highly dependent upon its conformation (¶15). In the Bach boiling method, potentization, which can only proceed in the cooling phase[10b], depends on the utilization of stored $\acute{\varepsilon}$ particles as a source of energy (¶11). They may be viewed as a type of static electricity, though with each particle only possessing a small fraction of the charge of an electron. Their main source is likely the magnetic field of -OH groups, which are themselves polarized and responsible for hydrogen bonding.

15a Another important issue is the ability of a vessel of circular section to act as a 'gravitational filter', preventing the ingress of extraneous patterns from external objects which might interfere with the development of an accurate 'cast'[10a]. It does this by rendering any such obtrusive gravitation spatially chaotic, which even includes any such resulting from its own structure[15b]. However, with both active and passive electromagnetic potentizers, the situation is a little more complicated, since two vessels are involved, one enclosing the other. The fixed outer wall is metallic (usually brass) and receives pattern information via a magnetic field; and the removable inner one, which contains the recipient, is usually made of either plastic or glass. Although both cylindrical vessels function as 'gravitational filters', the inner one allows the ingress of pattern information carried by electromagnetism. Nevertheless, if the inner vessel were made of a strongly ferromagnetic material (which is an unlikely situation), then this would most likely interfere with the correct processing of the recipient.

15b There is another, slightly more complex, way of looking at gravitational filtration. In any homoeopathic gravitational filtration system, the ability of the vessel to modify extraneous gravitational patterning appears to be related to the geometric constraints of circularity. The circle possesses the property that any given length of segment (arc) always carries the same degree of angularity (>0 degrees) as any other of the same length, irrespective of its position. This is not the case with polygons (here loosely taken to include anything of three sides or more), where some linear segments carry different degrees of angularity from others; which must be the case for the shape to exist at all. Circularity thus implies continuous angular uniformity (>0 degrees), and we might postulate, in contrast, that 'intelligible' homoeopathic patterning itself is manifest in the form of polydimensional polyhedral (flat-faced) Euclidian arrangements of compressed space (or space-time), a polyhedron being the three-dimensional extension of a polygon. The preparatory vessel imposes significant (small radius) circularity on extraneous gravitational patterns, which then, because of their acquired continuous angular uniformity, become 'unrecognizable'; this being so, even when they are superimposed upon the homoeopathic spatial compressive patterns themselves. Since gravity is such a relatively weak force (although it appears strong in relation to very large bodies), the only significant intrusive gravitational effect is that which relates to the preparatory vessel (unless we were to pursue our potentization inside one of the great pyramids of Egypt, or any other massive angulated structure). The vessel, as I have implied, deals with itself. As for the general gravitational field of the Earth, which is by far the strongest, paradoxically it affects patterning only negligibly, if at all. This results from the fact that its own patterning is extremely coarse, so that a significant change in the pattern of spatial contraction caused by it can only be detected over many metres. Since the vial and its contents occupy such a small area, there is essentially no pattern to be excluded.

16a Distortions of hyperspace produced by such *excluded substances* are restricted to the *chaotic* zones of 'group casts' and do not contribute to patterning ($\Lambda=0$)[10a]. Exclusion would seem to be dependent upon conflicting hyperspatial imagery between one or more -H atoms and one or more -OH groups, but only where the rest of the molecule is either unopposed to this disharmony, or, as is the case with water, completely absent. The *general formula* for molecules which are so excluded appears to be $C_vO_w(CO)_xH_y(OH)_z$, irrespective of isotopic composition; where either v or w is an integer *or* zero; x must be *zero*; and y and z must both be *integers* and *not zero*. With regard to the OH^- ion, which can be expressed as $C_0O_0(CO)_0H_0(OH^-)_1$, since y=0, it is *not* excluded. Water itself is $C_0O_0(CO)_0H_1(OH)_1$, and *is* excluded (except with respect to the OH^- component of its minor, and essentially insignificant, dissociated form $H_3O^+OH^-$), as are ethanol (ethyl alcohol) $C_2O_0(CO)_0H_5(OH)_1$, other alcohols (but not phenols, since the -OH group is dissociated in solution), lactose $\{C_{12}O_3(CO)_0H_{14}(OH)_8 \pm C_0O_0(CO)_0H_1(OH)_1\}$, other disaccharides (e.g. sucrose), oligosaccharides (e.g. verbascose and lycopose) and polysaccharides (cellulose, that highly insoluble and major constituent of the cell walls of all higher plants, is thus not 'potentizable' even by means of trituration in the initial phases of the LM technique). Organic acids and esters are *not* excluded because of the presence of the carbonyl group $>C=O$ ($w>0$). This exerts a strong organizational influence upon hyperspatial architecture, and one which is quite sufficient to negate the chaotic effect of the -H versus -OH conflict[16b]. Terpenes, the major constituents of essential oils, are also not excluded, since they lack -OH groups (z=0) and hence the conflict. Moreover, all substances containing elements other than C, H or O, either exclusively or in combination with any of these, are potentially 'potentizable'.

16b There are a number of molecules which, despite the presence of carbonyl groups, may still be subject to *exclusion* (which we may term *circumstantially excluded substance*). These are monosaccharides, such as glucose and fructose, which are *non-topologically* continually pleomorphic; i.e. in solution they constantly change between linear and cyclic forms by the opening and closing of carbon rings. Whilst the linear form exhibits a carbonyl group, this is absent in the cyclic isomers. In other words, their geometry is highly unstable and results in *chaotic* rather than geometric distortion of hyperspace. In calculations of $\boldsymbol{\Psi}$ (relative concentration), therefore, their concentration, if significant, must be subtracted from the denominator[10a]. In the traditional potentization of, for example, a fruit juice, the presence of fructose will not influence the geometry of the remedy. However, it is possible to potentize such substances out of solution by initial trituration with lactose[22a]. Linear glucose, for example, could be effectively processed in this manner, perhaps up to 3c, after which potentization could be continued in the liquid phase in accordance with the principle outlined in ¶20. Indeed, this is one of the reasons, albeit minor, why LM potencies can be different from those prepared in the more usual manner from mother tincture.

16c Interestingly enough, high potencies (above D30) appear to be inactivated by exposure to non-patterned magnetic fields of 50 Hz for 15 minutes (Dana Ullman, 1995: see Benveniste). There are also experimental indications (Benveniste, 2001) that 'water memory' of histamine may be transferred to a computer and then transmitted with effect. There has been a suggestion that this involves the recording of specific frequencies. However, I am of the opinion that whatever electromagnetic waves are recorded are merely the *carriers* for geometrical patterning information in a different spatial system, this becoming associated supra-dimensionally with the digital information registered upon the disk. Thus, the particular frequencies involved are irrelevant (my full objection to the frequency hypothesis is to be found in Lessell, 1994: Element VIII). Furthermore, *in vitro* experimentation of this type bears little relation to what happens *in vivo*, where the mode of action of remedies is often quite different. In this regard, it is interesting to note that, according to some researchers (Milgrom, 2001: see Ennis), potentized histamine acts in a similar manner to material histamine upon basophil degranulation *in vitro*; whereas anecdotal clinical evidence suggests that they have *opposing* pharmaceutical actions *in vivo* (as is the usual case with homoeopathic remedies). All rather confusing, until we realise that such experiments involve the use of isolated cells rather than a whole living organism[16d], the electromagnetic field strengths of which differs considerably. Indeed, as soon as cells are extracted from an animal or human, they exhibit only their small contribution to the total field of the organism. The importance of this is that the potentized drug, unlike its material counterpart, acts primarily upon the 'aural field (¶27)', dependent for its strength upon the electromagnetic field[27a], and its effects are quite opposite according to the robustness or fragility of the latter (¶31). In this respect, it will also be apparent that the electromagnetic field strength of isolated cells will also vary according to their vigour, and also, thus, according to that of the organism from which they were derived, or what might be termed its 'constitution'; not to mention the nature of the medium in which they are suspended and the electromagnetic status of the laboratory environment. Hence, we might envisage that isolated cells of strong constitution or health under 'ideal' experimental conditions might not act consistently with current findings favourable to homoeopathy, and produce failure of experimental corroboration.

[16d] There is also some *in vitro* experimental evidence that biological non-cellular preparations may be influenced by potentized substances (Benveniste, 2001). Here we cannot invoke any explanation involving the electromagnetic field of living cells, and it must be emphasized that this effect is not likely connected with the way remedies act in the clinical situation. Furthermore, it is currently claimed that the potentized substance generally simulates the material form in such studies. For this to occur, the primary interaction must be directly between the pattern contained in 'water memory' and the inverted pattern of the receptor molecule contained in its own supra-dimensions[11a]; especially since it is extremely improbable that potentized water can take part directly in the normal physical aspect of chemical interaction[30a]. This 'supra-dimensional bonding', which is restricted to biological systems, most probably should be regarded as a test-tube phenomenon. Here again we might claim that the circularity of the vial has something to do with the whole business (¶15).

[21a] Apart from the blurring caused by previous geometric information written in the memory, there is also that caused by *chaotic information* transferred at the time of imprinting. As has been suggested, the proportion of chaotic or incoherent primary space present in a 'group cast' (and thus chaotic information in the donor image) is dependent upon the relative concentrations of the components of initial substance and any contaminants[10a]. This chaotic information forms a 'fog' which overlays the transferred pattern, as a result of which the lesser elements are rendered indiscernible. In consequence, they cannot be 'resonantly' enhanced or amplified by the process of serial potentization, and effectively disappear; which is yet another mechanism by which minor molecules or ions become deprived of any contribution to the ultimate geometry of the remedy. The process of developing potency is akin to image-intensification, but what

image results is dependent on the coherence or intelligibility of the information originally supplied. The greater the level of chaotic 'fog', the greater the likelihood of distortion or simplification of the image.

22a It is generally held that water is the key substance involved in homoeopathic memorization. Nevertheless, it could be sensibly postulated that any *excluded substance*[16a], such as ethanol or lactose, should demonstrate similar ability. For, it would seem that the very properties of a molecule that determine its *exclusion* are the very *same* as those necessary for *molecular memory*. In essence, any molecule whose 'cast' is totally *chaotic*[10a], is capable of both receiving and *retaining* intelligible geometric information (but see below[22b]). If non-excluded molecules do have any memory, which they must in a sense, then it is only of *themselves* and no other[11a,16a]. Only a molecule whose memory of itself is chaotic (non-patterned) has the potential to memorize the patterns of others. As has been suggested, the origin of exclusion is the gravitational or hyperspatial compressive conflict between -H atoms and -OH groups; and it may be inferred that it is this that confers the phenomenon of molecular memory. Water itself is the most important substance in this respect because of an unusual atomic configuration which gives rise to utter hyperspatial chaos. Firstly, being essentially a bifurcate -OH group (H–O–H) and nothing else, it has no 'molecular appendage' to negate the chaos created by the conflict. Secondly, this chaos is further exacerbated by the confusion of the roles of its two -H atoms. Each -H atom is both independent of and part of the -OH group at apparently the same time, thus even conflicting with itself. I say *apparently*, since, on quantum grounds, the role of the -H atoms in the 'construction' of the -OH group is more likely in a state of constant alternation. Nevertheless, so rapid would this alternation be, that the overall effect would be one of complete blurring of hyperspatial imagery. This situation is, therefore, even more chaotic than that which occurs with regard to lactose, ethanol and other excluded substances; for here, the relevant conflicting -H atoms are not involved in the formation of the oppositional -OH groups. Furthermore, whilst we may assume that the remainder of each molecule or 'molecular appendage' is too 'weak' to negate the chaos generated by the conflict, there remains the distinct possibility that it might be even more desirable for it to be totally absent, as is the case with water. In other words, there is probably always some geometric influence upon chaotic space produced by 'molecular appendages', albeit relatively insignificant with regard to excluded substances. Upon the basis of these arguments, it would seem likely that donor images are, indeed, transferred directly to the lactose molecule itself during trituration, with the bonded and unbonded water molecules playing but a small part in the process. Similarly, it would appear that ethanol plays almost as an important role in the retention of donor image as water itself. More remarkably, perhaps, we might conclude that the facility for molecular memory is more widespread in the world of chemistry than might have hitherto been thought.

22b Molecules, such as fructose and glucose, which are *circumstantially excluded substances*[16b], are not included in this concept. Any molecular memory they may acquire is likely lost at each of the frequent transformations from one isomeric state to another (linear, five-membered ring, six-membered ring). Furthermore, despite the fact that the cyclic forms appear to have the appropriate atomic configuration for exhibiting molecular memory, the linear form (in that it contains a carbonyl group) does not. In other words, whereas they might be capable of receiving information, they have no means of retaining it.

26a There are some unusual remedies in homoeopathy initially prepared by exposing glass vials containing ethanol–water to various types of radiation or to magnetic fields for varying lengths of time (which are then subjected to normal serial potentization). These include: Sol (Sunlight), Luna (Moonlight), X-ray, VDU and Magnetis polus australis (South pole of the magnet). Since such things, being immaterial, do not, in themselves, displace primary space, it would seem inconsistent that remedies might be made from them. However, they can influence the behaviour of the electrons of the water (or ethanol[22a]) molecule and thus alter its physical characteristics. In order to give some sensible explanation to this phenomenon, it is useful to consider the electron as being a ball composed of a thread-like string[8b] wound around a notional axis; this, for the sake of illustration, pointing, say, towards the centre of gravity of the atom, located in the nuclear space (this, of course, goes against the quantum dogma that electrons, as with other leptons, are without substructure). The effect of introducing an extraneous radiation or magnetic field is to alter the angle of this axis, so that it no longer points towards the atomic centre of gravity. The degree of angulation from the 'norm' will be determined by the nature of the source of influence (i.e. frequency or magnetic field characteristics), and will be unique to it. Since the electronic strings are now aligned differently with respect to the nucleus, the water molecule is thus modified and its distortion of primary space altered; although the effect of 'angular perturbation', as we might call it, is rather feeble, with only a small patterning influence on the normal spatial chaos of the 'cast' surrounding the molecule (for, if it were great, then water, rather like most other molecules, would no longer have any memory function capable of potentization or enhancement[22a]). Nevertheless, as a result of this, it becomes an image donor to itself[11a] or other water molecules. However, where such radiation (as in Bach solar energization) or magnetism (as in a Rae card-pattern potentizer) is involved in the production of another remedy, so weak is the angular perturbation effect that it would seem that any spatial patterning it might have produced is annihilated. Another point of interest is that sunlight *slowly* de-potentizes homoeopathic remedies, but only in the higher potencies where the original substance is absent. In the lower potencies, where there is still the significant presence of the donor, it encourages potentization. If this were not the case, there would be no Bach Flower Remedies, other than those prepared by boiling. Sunlight achieves the de-potentization of higher potencies by a combination of the angular perturbation effect of UV light upon valency-shell electrons and its ability to supply adequate energy to the system. In this manner, any pre-existing information held in the supra-dimensional memory system of the recipient (water or ethanol) becomes overwritten with that concerning UV light itself.

[27a] In reality, the aural field (AF) is fundamentally composed of the aggregate of the supra-dimensional 'memory fields' (MF) of the molecules which comprise the body. It has already been proposed that all molecules have such fields[11a]. The overall three-dimensional spatial system occupied by the MF and the AF is, indeed, one and the same. Since animals and plants are dominantly composed of water, the bulk of the AF is derived from its MF. In its natural state, the MF of water is essentially devoid of patterning information[22a], additionally limited by the stringent requirements for potentization (potentization is essentially an *in vitro* process, and even though it may occur to an extremely limited degree within the pipes of a water delivery system or bottles, such water, when entering the cells, makes little impression on the AF). An AF largely based on the MF of water is thus free to gather and process new information (as with RAM in a computer). We may conceptualize the AF as being composed of a higher dimensional field of magnetism (¶16). It is thus fairly simple to see how the higher dimensions of the conventionally measurable electromagnetic field of the body and the fundamental AF can interact. This combinative association becomes what is known as the 'vital force' (the Chinese word *Qi* embraces this concept

together with the more conventional aspects of bodily electromagnetism). Viewed in projection into our normal physical space, this extends for a short distance outside the bounds of the material body to form an *aura*, where it may be influenced by various phenomena (e.g. meteorological static), personal contact and medical techniques. When the practitioner places a hand very close to, or directly upon, a patient, there is an overlap of the auras of both parties. Some subjects are so sensitive, that merely having a vial containing potentized homoeopathic material placed in close proximity to them will produce a noticeable effect. This has been shown even with tadpoles (Dana Ullman, 1995: see Endler et al.). Again, the projective aura of the remedy extends outside the normal physical boundaries of the vessel in which it is contained.

[30a] Many, but not all, drugs (or toxins) work by their interaction with chemical receptor sites. In order for this to occur, the receptor must have an electrochemical affinity with the drug; that is to say, some form of chemical bonding must be possible. All known types of interaction have been described: ionic, van der Waals', hydrogen and even covalent[16d]. Effectively, a new entity is produced, viz. a chemical compound of the drug plus the receptor. However, both the drug and the receptor, and indeed their unified complex, are immersed in the electromagnetic field of the body. Idiosyncratic drug resistance (unresponsiveness) may be at least partially explained by the interference of this field with the zone around the receptor, so as to alter its electromagnetic status, and thus its affinity. Alternatively, bonding does occur, but the electromagnetic configuration of the drug-receptor complex, or that of any consequential chemical interaction, is opposed by that of the body. In homoeopathy, we would call this a 'constitutional' influence on the ability of a drug to succeed or otherwise. Furthermore, at this level, homoeopathic remedies may well work by influencing the status of the body's background electromagnetic field[16c]. The action of a toxin such as mercury may be blocked by sufficiently modifying this field, so that bonding is no longer possible at the receptor site; with the subsequent release of the toxin and its excretion. Under other circumstances, the modified background field may combine with the electrochemical field of the receptor to simulate the presence of a drug or something with an inverted electromagnetic pattern[30b]. Ultimately, it is the change in electromagnetic pattern of the receptor which induces subsequent physicochemical changes in the body; and this, as has been stated, may be induced by the action of a drug or, even without one, by the influence of the body's electromagnetic field suitably altered by homoeopathy. It is also worth stating that the increased risk of leukaemia in those subjected to the magnetic field of overhead power lines illustrates the relevance of electromagnetism in the development of disease or otherwise. As any drug receptor is immersed in the electromagnetic field of the body, so the body itself is immersed in that of the environment. Is it, therefore, not surprising to learn that some people are actually worse before thunder storms, and better afterwards; or that the electrical status of the environment can determine the efficacy or otherwise of either a drug or a homoeopathic remedy?

[30b] Interestingly enough, ordinary drug molecules must carry a negative image of themselves in the appropriate dimensions of hyperspace[11a]. This, however, having not been subjected to intensification via potentization, is relatively weak in influence. Only in exceptional circumstances, where the patient has a peculiar sensitivity (derived from a type of constitutional sympathetic resonance with the negative image), does it produce a negation of drug-receptor interaction or an inverse effect at the receptor site. However, even with orthodox drugs, an inverse response is not unknown, whereby the patient on medication does the opposite of what is expected. Moreover, some cases of unresponsiveness may also result from something of this sort. Such a mechanism is indirect, firstly via the aural field, and then through the electromagnetic.

References

(The internet sites are particularly valuable for information on quantum theories and general references)

Benveniste, Jacques (2001) *From 'Water Memory' Effects to 'Digital Biology'* http://www.digibio.com/

Dana Ullman (1995) *Scientific Evidence of Homeopathic Medicine*. Located at: http://www.homeopathic.com/research/scienti.htm

Gribbin, John (1999) *Q is for Quantum*. Phoenix Giant (a brilliantly written reference book on modern theoretical and experimental physics)

Lessell, Colin B (1994). *The Infinitesimal Dose*. Daniel, C.W. ed., (a thorough description of most physical hypotheses of homoeopathic pharmacy hitherto proposed, together with many references)

Milgrom, L. (2001) *Thanks for the Memory*. The Guardian, Thursday 15th March 2001. Also via Brian Josephson's homepage: http://www.tcm.phy.cam.ac.uk/~bdj10/

Appendix 4

List of professional suppliers

(with international mail order facilities)

The following is only a brief list, and there are many other reliable suppliers:

Herbal medicines

Phyto Products Ltd, Park Works, Park Road, Mansfield Woodhouse, Mansfield, Notts NG19 8ED, UK
Tel: 01623 644334; fax: 01623 657232; e-mail: info@phyto.co.uk

Nutritional supplements

Lamberts Healthcare Ltd, Lamberts Road, Tunbridge Wells, Kent TN2 3EH, UK
Tel: 01892 554313; fax: 01892 515863

Pharma Nord Aps, Sadelmagervej 30-32, 7100 Vejle, Denmark
Tel: 7585 7400; fax: 7585 7474

Essential Sterolin Products (Pty) Ltd, 16th Road, Randjespark, Midrand 1685, South Africa [manufacturers of Moducare™]
E-mail (USA/Canada): info@moducare.com
E-mail (UK): moducare@iafrica.com

Homoeopathic remedies, Bach Flower Remedies, reference books

Ainsworth's Homoeopathic Pharmacy, 36 New Cavendish Street, London W1G 8UF, UK
Tel: 020 7935 5330; fax: 020 7486 4313

Helios Homoeopathic Pharmacy, 97 Camden Road, Tunbridge Wells, Kent TN1 2QR, UK
Tel: 01892 536393/537254; fax: 01892 546850

Homeopathic Educational Services, 2124 Kittredge Street, Berkeley, CA 94704, USA
Tel: (510) 649 0294/(800) 359 9051; fax: (510) 649 1955
E-mail: mail@homeopathic.com

Hahnemann Laboratories Inc, 1940 Fourth Street, San Rafael, CA 94901, USA
Tel: 1 888 4 ARNICA/1 888 427 6422; fax: 1 415 451 6981

Brauer Biotherapies (Pty) Ltd, Para Road, Adelaide 5000, Australia
Tel: (0) 8 8563 2932; fax: (0) 8 8563 3398

Index of Medicaments

Nutritional supplements

S-adenosylmethionine (SAM), Gilbert's syndrome 122
Alpha Lipoic Acid, glaucoma (adjunctive therapy) 123
Anthocyanadin complex *see* Colladeen

Benecol, high LDL cholesterol 87
Bioflavanoids, menorrhagia 156
Borage Oil
  amputation pain, if diabetic 62
  Bell's palsy 74
  burning foot syndrome 81
  diabetic neuropathy 101
  dyslexia 105
  dyspraxia 106
  multiple sclerosis 160

Calcium
  coeliac disease 89
  pregnancy 180
Calcium pantothenate, burning foot syndrome 81
Caprylic acid, chronic gastrointestinal candidiasis 83
L-Carnitine
  atrial fibrillation 70
  Raynaud's disease 185
Cherries, gout prevention 124
Chitosan
  hypertension 134
  obesity 167
Chondroitin sulphate
  high LDL cholesterol 87
  osteoarthritis 169
  Scheuermann's disease 192
Chromium
  cravings for sweet things 94
  hypoglycaemia 135
Citrus Bioflavonoids, gingivitis and periodontitis 123
Cod Liver Oil
  bedsores 73
  cataracts 85
  osteoarthritis 169
  osteoporosis 170
Coenzyme Q10
  angina prevention 64
  asthma 69
  chronic sinusitis 196
  gingivitis and periodontitis 123
  hay fever 128
  heart disease 130
  hypertension 134
  male infertility 140
  premature ventricular beats 180
Colladeen
  capillary fragility 83
  cataracts 85
  diabetic retinopathy 101
  Eales' disease 107
  fibromyalgia 116
  macular degeneration 153
  night blindness 165
  varicose cellulitis 85

Commiphora mukul,
hypertriglyceridaemia 208

Diabetes mellitus nutritional support cocktail 100
Digestive enzymes, Crohn's disease 95

Evening Primrose Oil
fibrocystic breast disease 115
Raynaud's disease 185

Flax Seed Oil
arthritis 68, 69
atherosclerosis 69
atrophic vaginitis 212
cancer support 83
dyslexia 105
dysmenorrhoea 105
dyspraxia 106
eczema, internal therapy 107
hypertension 134
hypertriglyceridaemia 208
lupus erythematosus (adjunctive therapy) 210
menopausal hot flushes 156
migraine prevention 157
multiple sclerosis 160
nephrotic syndrome 163
paranoid schizophrenia 192
psoriasis 182
Raynaud's disease 185
tremor 208
ulcerative colitis 209
varicose cellulitis 85
varicose veins 213
Florisene, alopecia 61
Folic acid
Alzheimer's disease 62
coeliac disease 89
idiopathic vitiligo 215
pregnancy 180
ulcerative colitis 209

Garlic Extract
hypertension 134
hypertriglyceridaemia 208
Raynaud's disease 185
Glucosamine sulphate
athletic support 70
carpal tunnel syndrome 84
chondromalacia patellae 88
dislocations 103
frozen shoulder 195
ganglia 121
lumbago 151
osteoarthritis 169
Scheuermann's disease 192
sciatica 192
sprains 198
tennis elbow 203
L-Glutamine, food allergy 118

Hesperidin, menopausal hot flushes 156
Hydroxocobalamin *see* Vitamin B12

Iron
anaemia 63
coeliac disease 89

Kérastase Système Détox Shampooing Antipelliculaire, dandruff 98

Lecithin
chronic hepatitis 131
eczema 108

Lycopersicon esculentum extract, asthma 69
L-lysine, aphthous ulcers 67

Magnesium
attention deficit-hyperactivity disorder 70
coeliac disease 89
dysmenorrhoea 105
fracture union 119
glaucoma (adjunctive therapy) 123
hypoglycaemia 135
premenstrual syndrome 180
valvular heart disease 130
Manganese, tardive dyskinesia 202
Methyl Sulphonyl Methane (MSM)
brittle nails 162
cancer support 83
chronic blepharitis 76
chronic bronchitis 79
eczema, internal therapy 107
Moducare
arthritis 68
Behçets disease 74
cancer support 82
eczema, internal therapy 107
Grave's disease (adjunctive therapy) 124
idiopathic thrombocytopenic purpura 183

lupus erythematosus (adjunctive therapy) 210
nephrotic syndrome 163
polymyalgia rheumatica (adjunctive therapy) 179
primary hypothyroidism 135
proctitis 181
prostate hypertrophy 181
ulcerative colitis 209
MSM *see* Methyl Sulphonyl Methane
Multivitamin-mineral supplement, AIDS 59

NADH (nicotinamide adenine dinucleotide)
Alzheimer's disease 62
Parkinson's disease 174
postviral syndrome 179

Organic sulphur *see* Methyl Sulphonyl Methane
Osteogard, osteoporosis 170

Pancreatic enzymatic supplements, chronic pancreatitis 174
Pantothenic Acid
chronic sinusitis 196
hay fever 128
L-Phenylalanine, idiopathic vitiligo 215
Phosphatidyl choline
chronic hepatitis 131
eczema 108

Phytomenadione
morning sickness 159
osteoporosis 171

Royal Jelly, high LDL cholesterol 87

SAM (S-adenosylmethionine), Gilbert's syndrome 122
Selenium, Osgood-Schlatter's disease 169
Shitake Extract, chronic hepatitis 131
Spirulina fusiformis, oral leukoplakia 149

Vitamin A
coeliac disease 89
menorrhagia 156
night blindness 165
Vitamin B complex
alcoholic neuritis 164
alcoholism, liver protection 60
cirrhosis of the liver 88
Vitamin B1
mosquito bite prevention 75
poor memory 155
Vitamin B2, angular cheilitis 65
Vitamin B6
carpal tunnel syndrome 84
coeliac disease 89
fluid retention 117
monosodium glutamate sensitivity 87
morning sickness 159
polymyalgia rheumatica (adjunctive therapy) 179
poor memory 155
premenstrual syndrome 180
Vitamin B12, idiopathic vitiligo 215
Vitamin B12 (hydroxocobalamin) *see* injections: Vitamin B12 (hydroxocobalamin)
Vitamin C
bedsores 73
common colds 90
high LDL cholesterol 87
idiopathic vitiligo 215
male infertility 140
menopausal hot flushes 156
menorrhagia 156
morning sickness 159
wound healing 217
Vitamin D, coeliac disease 89
Vitamin E
angina prevention 64
atherosclerosis 69
burns and scalds 81
cataracts 85
diabetes mellitus nutritional support 100
fibrocystic breast disease 115
haemorrhoids 126
herpes simplex 131
high LDL cholesterol 87
infertility 140
menopausal hot flushes 156
menorrhagia 156
oral leukoplakia 149
Osgood-Schlatter's disease 169
premenstrual syndrome 180
tardive dyskinesia 202
varicose veins 213
yellow nail syndrome 163
Vitamin E cream
scars 191
sunburn 200

Vitamin K, coeliac disease 89
Vitamin-mineral cocktail, athletic support 70

Zinc
acne vulgaris 57
alopecia 61
anorexia and bulimia nervosa 65
bedsores 73
brittle nails 162
chocolate cravings 94
coeliac disease 89
common colds 90
fracture union 119
giardiasis 122
glandular fever 123
loss of smell and taste 197
male infertility 140
night blindness 165
postviral syndrome 179
pregnancy 180
presbycusis 180
prostate hypertrophy 181
recurrent boils 77
tinnitus 206
white spots on nails 163
Wilson's disease 216
wound healing 217
Zinc monoglycerate/sulphate cream, herpes simplex 131

❀ Herbal medicines

Aesculus hippocastanum
phlebitis 177
varicose veins 213
Agropyron repens, cystitis 97
Aloë vera gel
burns and scalds 81
callus calcis 82
lichen planus 149
psoriasis 182
seborrhoeic dermatitis 193
sunburn 200
Anal fissures, cream for 63
Arnica montana
acute sprain 198
bruises 80

Barosma betulina, cystitis 97
Berberis aquifolium, callus calcis 82
Bunion cream 80

Calendula officinalis
abrasions 56
Bartholin's abscess and cyst 73
blisters 76
chaps 86
chickenpox 86
corns 93
cracked lips 150
sore nipples 165
wounds 217
Capsaicin, neuralgia 164
Carduus marianus
alcoholism, liver protection 60
cirrhosis of the liver 88
gallstones 121
Gilbert's syndrome 122
hepatitis 130
Castor oil purge, tapeworm 202
Chilblain cream 87
Cinnamomum zeylanicum
chronic gastrointestinal candidiasis 83
menorrhagia 156
Citronella Oil, mosquito bite prevention 75
Commiphora molmol
gingivitis and periodontitis 123
herpes simplex 131
Commiphora mukul, obesity 167
Crataegus oxycanthoides
amoebiasis 62
angina prevention 64
Crohn's disease 95
diarrhoea 65, 102
diverticulitis 103
giardiasis 122
hiatus hernia 132
irritable bowel syndrome 143
overindulgence 172
viral gastroenteritis 122
Curcurbita pepo, tapeworm 202

Delphinium staphisagria, head-lice 128
Dhobi's itch, cream for 100
Dimethyl sulphoxide (DMSO) gel
cutaneous amyloidosis 63
Dupuytren's contracture 104
Peyronie's disease 177
reflex sympathetic dystrophy 106
scleroderma 192
Dr Zhao's Fabao 101D™ formula lotion, alopecia 61

Echinacea angustifolia
acute sinusitis 196
boils 77
cancer support 83
carbuncles 83
corneal ulcers 93
diverticulitis 103
granuloma annulare 124
herpes simplex prevention 131
influenza 141
viral gastroenteritis 122
Wegener's granulomatosis 216
Eczema cream 108
Eye-drops
cataracts 84
conjunctivitis 92
corneal ulcers *see* eye-drops: conjunctivitis
herpes zoster *see* eye drops: conjunctivitis

Feverfew, migraine prevention 157

Ginkgo biloba
Alzheimer's disease 61
asthma 69
atherosclerosis 69
chronic bronchitis 79
chronic sinusitis 196
diabetic retinopathy 101
Eales' disease 107
hay fever 128
impotence 138
macular degeneration 153
migraine prevention 157
poor memory 155
presbycusis 180
tinnitus 205
Ginseng *see* Panax ginseng
Glycyrrhiza glabra
eczema 108
insect bites and stings 75
Grapefruit Seed Extract (GSE), amoebiasis 62
Griffonia Bean Extract
anxiety and depression 66
fibromyalgia 116
insomnia 142
jet lag 145
obesity 167
postnatal depression 179
tinnitus 205
Gum guggulu
hypertriglyceridaemia 208
obesity 167

Gymnema sylvestre, diabetes mellitus (adjunctive therapy) 100

Hamamelis virginiana, eczema 108
Harpagophytum procumbens
gout 124
polymyalgia rheumatica (adjunctive therapy) 179
Head-lice formula 128
Hops powder, insomnia 142
Hypericum perforatum
anorexia and bulimia nervosa 65
anxiety 66, 115
bereavement 74
depression 66
postnatal 179
seasonal affective disorder 190
epilepsy (adjunctive therapy) 110
obsessive-compulsive disorder 167
paranoia 174
paranoid schizophrenia 192
phobias 177
agoraphobia 59
claustrophobia 89
premature ejaculation 180

Impatiens capensis, poison ivy/oak rash 178
Impetigo cream 138

Jasmine Oil, aphrodisiac 66
Jewelweed, poison ivy/oak rash 178

Khellin, vitiligo 215

Lavender Oil
eczema 108
otitis externa 171
Lemon Oil, verruca 214
Liriosma ovata
diminished libido 149
impotence 138

Mahonia aquifolium, psoriasis 182
Muira Puama
diminished libido 149
impotence 138
Myrrh
gingivitis and periodontitis 123
herpes simplex 131

Neem Oil, head-lice 128, 129
Neem Oil cream
  athlete's foot 70
  Dhobi's itch 100
  pityriasis versicolor 178
  ringworm 189
  scabies 191
Nicotine patches, ulcerative colitis 209

Panax ginseng
  adrenal depletion 58
  diabetes mellitus (adjunctive therapy) 100
  postviral syndrome 179
Papain, jellyfish stings 145
Peuraria lobata, alcohol cravings 60
Picrasma excelsa, head-lice 128
Pine Bark Extract *see* Pycnogenol
Plantago major
  post-extraction osteitis 104
  sensitive teeth 202
Plantago psyllium, constipation 92
Propolis
  aphthous ulcers 67
  atrophic vaginitis 212
  Behçet's disease 74
  folliculitis 118
  hand, foot and mouth disease 127
  impetigo 138
  ingrowing toenails 141
  molluscum contagiosum 158
  paronychia 175
  post-extraction osteitis 104
Pycnogenol
  atrial fibrillation 70
  capillary fragility 83
  chickenpox 87
  psoriasis 182
PZ cream
  bunions 80
  carpal tunnel syndrome *see* PZ cream: bunions
  fibrositis *see* PZ cream: bunions
  osteoarthritis *see* PZ cream: bunions
  shin splints *see* PZ cream: bunions

Quercus spp. decoction, eczema 108

Rosmarinus officinalis, chickenpox 86
Ruscus aculeatus, lymphoedema post-mastectomy 152

Salix alba
  general analgesia 64, 129
  migraine prevention 157
  osteoarthritis 170
Schoenenberger Plant Juice *see* Tussilago farfara folia
Scutellaria lateriflora, epilepsy (adjunctive therapy) 110
Serenoa serrulata
  alopecia 61
  prostatitis 181
Siberian ginseng
  adrenal depletion 58
  postviral syndrome 179
Slippery Elm, ulcerative colitis 209
Smilax spp.
  acne vulgaris 57
  barber's itch 73
  callus calcis 82
  chronic blepharitis 76
  psoriasis 182
  rosacea 189
  seborrhoeic dermatitis 193
Stellaria media, dhobi's itch 100
Syrupus Ficorum, constipation 92
Syzygium jambolanum
  diabetes mellitus (adjunctive therapy) 100
  diabetic retinopathy 101

Tamus communis fructus, chilblains 87
Tea Tree Oil
  cradle cap 94
  dhobi's itch 100
  impetigo 138
  nails, fungal infections 162
  paronychia 175
  trichomonas vaginitis 212–13
  verruca 214
Tea Tree Oil cream
  athlete's foot 70
  ringworm 189
Thuja occidentalis, verruca 214
Triple Rose-Water
  abrasions 56
  balanitis 72
  incisional abscesses 56
  infection of mastoid cavity 154
Tussilago farfara folia
  acute bronchitis 79
  acute tracheitis 207
  common dry cough 94

Ulmus fulva/rubra powder, ulcerative colitis 209
Urtica dioica/urens
  flight oedema 168
  fluid retention 117
  gout 124
  heat oedema of ankles 130
  inadequate lactation 147
  solar urticaria 200

Valerian powder, insomnia 142
Verruca formula 214
Vinegar, jellyfish stings 145
Viola tricolor, dhobi's itch 100
Vitamin E Oil, trichomonas vaginitis 212-13
Vitex agnus-castus
  acne vulgaris 57
  atrophic vaginitis 212
  dysmenorrhoea 105
  female infertility 140
  fibrocystic breast disease 115
  fluid retention 117
  menopausal hot flushes 156
  menorrhagia 156
  osteoarthritis 170
  osteoporosis 171
  polycystic ovary syndrome 178
  premenstrual syndrome 180

Zea mays
  chronic prostatitis 181
  cystitis 97
  enuresis 110
  renal calculi, prevention 82
Zingiber officinalis
  acute sinusitis 196
  arthritis 68
  common colds 90
  dyspepsia 105
  fibrositis 116
  Helicobacter pylori infection 130
  migraine prevention 157
  morning/motion sickness 159
  osteoarthritis 169
  sore throat 197
  viral gastroenteritis 122

✕ Homoeopathic remedies

ABC 30c, infantile fever 115
Abrotanum, hydrocele 134
Acidum benzoicum, gout 124
Acidum fluoricum, fistulae 117
Acidum muriaticum
  Ménière's disease 155
  vertigo 214
Acidum nitricum
  acute necrotizing ulcerative gingivitis 122
  anal fissures 63
  ecthyma contagiosum 107
Acidum phosphoricum
  alopecia 60
  glandular fever 123
Acidum salicylicum, Ménière's disease 155
Acidum sulphuricum, chronic urticaria 211
Aconite
  anticipatory anxiety 66
  Bell's palsy 74
  croup 96
  epistaxis 110
  fright 119
  hypertension 134
  infantile fever 115
  stroke 200
Actaea racemosa
  abdominal pain 55
  fibrositis 116
Aesculus hippocastanum, haemorrhoids 126
Agaricus muscarius, frostbite 119
Agraphis nutans, otitis media 172
Allergens, allergies 60
Allium cepa
  hay fever 128
  pain following amputation 62
Ambra grisea, idiopathic pruritus 182
Ammi visnaga, steroidal vitiligo 215
Ammonium carbonicum
  acute bronchitis 79
  meningitis (adjunctive therapy) 156
Ammonium muriaticum, sciatica 192
Anthracinum, recurrent boils 77
Antimonium crudum, impetigo 138
Antimonium tartaricum
  acne vulgaris 57
  bronchitis 79
  chickenpox 87
  hand, foot and mouth disease 127
  impetigo 138
  pneumonia (adjunctive therapy) 178

Apis mellifica
  bursitis 81
  erythema nodosum 111
  scarlatina 191
Argentum metallicum, laryngitis 148
Argentum nitricum
  anticipatory anxiety 66
  conjunctivitis 92
  fear of heights 115
  headache 129
Arnica
  acute sprain 198
  anaesthesia, ill effects of local 63
  analgesia 64
  bruises 80
  haematoma 126
  haemorrhage 126
  lumbago 151
Arsenicum album
AIDS 59
  alopecia 60
  diarrhoea 102
  hay fever 128
  kala azar 146
  lichen planus 149
  lymphoedema of lower extremities 152
  pityriasis rosea 178
  psoriasis 182
  sciatica 192
  viral gastroenteritis 122
Arsenicum iodatum
  dhobi's itch 100
  psoriasis 182
Arum triphyllum, laryngitis 148
Aspergillus spp., aspergillosis 69
Aurum metallicum, valvular heart disease 130
Aurum muriaticum kalinatum, uterine fibroids 116
Aurum muriaticum natronatum
  undescended testes 204
  uterine fibroids 116

Bacillinum
  cervical lymphadenopathy 152
  coeliac disease 89
  dermatitis herpetiformis 99
  food desensitization 118
  prevention of influenza 141
  ringworm 189
  sarcoidosis 191
Baryta carbonica, tonsillar hypertrophy 206
Belladonna
  acute pancreatitis 174
  erythema infectiosum 111
  gallstones 121
  headache 129, 200
  infantile fever 115
  otitis media 171
  scarlatina 191
  varicose cellulitis 85
Bellis perennis
  abdominal pain 55
  lumbago 151
Berberis vulgaris, renal colic 90
Borax
  antibiotics, ill effects of 65
  barotrauma prevention 73
  noise intolerance 165
  thrush 205
Borrelia burgdorferi, Lyme disease prevention 151
Brucella abortus, brucellosis 80
Bryonia
  acute pleurisy 178
  cough 94
  erythema infectiosum 111
  pneumonia (adjunctive therapy) 178

Cactus grandiflorus, angina 64
Caeruleum methylenum, bilharzia prevention 75
Caladium, idiopathic pruritus 182
Calcarea carbonica
  acromegaly 57
  Ménière's disease 155
  otitis media 171
  ranula 185
  warts 216
Calcarea fluorica
  adhesions 58
  aneurysm 64
  ankylosing spondylitis 65
  dislocations 103
  Dupuytren's contracture 104
  Ehlers-Danlos syndrome 109
  frozen shoulder 195
  haemorrhoids 126
  heamangioma 126
  lax ligament syndrome 148
  lumbago 151
  Osgood-Schlatter's disease 169
  osteoma 170
  osteoporosis 171
  otosclerosis 172

salivary calculi 190
Scheuermann's disease 192
sialectasis 195
thyroid cysts, benign 97
valvular heart disease 130
Calcarea phosphorica
Osgood-Schlatter's disease 169
tonsillar hypertrophy 206
Calcarea renalis, dental calculus reduction 82
Candida albicans, chronic gastrointestinal candidiasis 83
Cannabis indica, multiple sclerosis 160
Cannabis sativa, urethral caruncle 210
Cantharis
acute cystitis 97
insect bites and stings 75
urethritis (adjunctive therapy) 210
Capsicum, homesickness 133
Carbo animalis, pain following pleurisy 178
Carbo vegetabilis
bedsores 73
collapse 90
eructation 111
Castor equi, sore nipples 165
Cat-scratch fever, cat-scratch fever 84
Caulophyllum, labour 147
Causticum
acute tracheitis 207
Bell's palsy 74
nerve trauma 163
stress incontinence 199
Chamomilla
aerodontalgia 59
anaesthesia, anxiety before local 63
immunization, prevention of adverse reactions 137
infantile colic 90
infantile fever 115
infantile temper tantrums 203
teething 203
Cheiranthus, pericoronitis 176
China officinalis
diarrhoea 102
haemorrhage 126
irritable bowel syndrome 143
malaria (adjunctive prevention) 153
viral gastroenteritis 122
Chlorinum, chlorine conjunctivitis prevention 92
Cholesterinum, gallstones 121
Chromium kali sulphuratum, hay fever 128
Chrysanthemum parthenium, aphthous ulcers 67
Cicuta virosa, meningitis (adjunctive therapy) 156
Cimicifuga racemosa
abdominal pain 55
fibrositis 116
Cina
infantile temper tantrums 203
threadworms 204
Clematis erecta
acute orchitis 169
chronic blepharitis 76
epididymitis 110
Coca, mountain sickness 159
Cocculus indicus
jet lag 145
motion sickness 159
Coccus cacti, removal of conjunctival foreign bodies 118
Coffea cruda
aerodontalgia 59
anticipatory anxiety 66
fear of joy 145
insomnia 142
Collinsonia canadensis, haemorrhoids 126
Colocynthis
dysmenorrhoea 105
infantile colic 90
sciatica 192
Conium maculatum, vertigo 214
Cuprum arsenitum, pain following amputation 62
Cuprum metallicum
cramp 94
whooping cough 216
Cyclamen, amenorrhoea 62

Desensitization to food, preparations for 118
Dioscorea villosa, gallstones 121
Drosera, whooping cough 216

E. coli, chronic prostatitis 181
Entamoeba histolytica, amoebiasis 62
Eupatorium perfoliatum, dengue 99
Euphrasia, conjunctivitis 92

Ferrum metallicum, headache 129

Ferrum phosphoricum
  epistaxis 110
  haemorrhage 126
Folliculinum, polycystic ovary syndrome 178
Fragaria, dental calculus reduction 82
Fraxinus Americana, uterine fibroids 116

Gelsemium
  anticipatory anxiety 66
  encephalitis 109
  influenza 141
  zombielike states 220
Glandular fever nosode, glandular fever 123
Gluten, coeliac disease 89
Gunpowder
  boils 77
  incisional abscesses 56
  paronychia 175

Hamamelis virginiana
  haemorrhoids 126
  phlebitis 177
Hecla lava
  dental cysts 96
  post-extraction osteitis 104
Hepar sulph.
  Bartholin's abscess and cyst 73
  corneal ulcers 93
  croup 96
  dental abscesses 56
  dental pulpitis 183
  dental focal sepsis, testing for 118
  pericoronitis 176
  quinsy 184
  uveitis (adjunctive therapy) 211
House Dust Mite, chronic sinusitis (mite allergy) 196
Hydrastis, aspergillosis 69
Hydrocotyle asiatica, psoriasis 182
Hydrocyanic acid, whooping cough 216
Hyoscyamus, delirium tremens 98
Hypericum
  coccidynia 89
  nerve trauma 163

Ignatia, tobacco smoke sensitivity 197
Influenzinum, prevention of influenza 141
Iodum, chronic pancreatitis 174
Ipecacuanha
  haemorrhage 126
  nausea after general anaesthesia 63
Iris tenax, acute appendicitis 67
Iris versicolor, migraine 158

Jaborandi, mumps 160
Jacaranda caroba, balanitis 72

Kali bichromicum, acute sinusitis 196
Kali bromatum, acne vulgaris 57
Kali carbonicum, warts 216
Kali iodatum
  acute sinusitis 196
  bursitis 81
Kali muriaticum
  barotrauma prevention 73
  otitis media 172
Kali phosphoricum
  adrenal depletion 58
  chronic hypotension 135
  postherpetic neuralgia 164
  weariness of mind 112
Kali sulphuricum, infection of mastoid cavity 154

Lac caninum, to stop lactation 147
Lachesis
  delirium tremens 98
  haemorrhage 126
  quinsy 184
Lachnantes, stiff neck 199
Lapis albus
  actinomycosis 58
  cervical lymphadenopathy 152
Latrodectus mactans, angina 64
Ledum
  acute sprains 198
  anaesthesia, discomfort after local 63
  black eyes 76
  insect bites and stings 75
Lueticum, osteoarthritis 170
Lycopodium
  brucellosis 80
  chronic prostatitis 181
Crohn's disease 95
  glaucoma (adjunctive therapy) 123
  irritable bowel syndrome 143
  renal colic 90

Magnesia phosphorica
  hiccups 132

influenza 141
sciatica 192
Magnetis polus australis, ingrowing toenails 141
Malaria officinalis, malaria (adjunctive prevention) 153
Medorrhinum
catarrh 85
chronic sinusitis 196
cystic fibrosis 97
otitis media 171
polycystic ovary syndrome 178
polyps 179
prevention of barotrauma 73
warts 216
Meningococcinum, meningitis (adjunctive therapy) 156
Mercurius corrosivus
acute cystitis 97
corneal ulcers 93
dysentery 105
sore throat 197
uveitis (adjunctive therapy) 211
Mercurius solubilis
acute necrotizing ulcerative gingivitis 122
AIDS 59
balanitis 72
multiple sclerosis 160
teething 203
Mezereum
head-lice 129
impetigo 138
Millefolium, haemorrhage 126
Mixed regional pollens/grasses, hay fever 128
Myristica
acute boils 77
dental abscesses 56

Natrum muriaticum
herpes simplex prevention 131
menopausal arthritis 68
postnatal depression 179
Sjögren's syndrome 196
Natrum salicylicum, Ménière's disease 155
Natrum sulphuricum
concussion 91
epilepsy (adjunctive therapy) 110
influenza 141
Nux vomica
hangovers 127
influenza 141
inguinal hernias 131
overindulgence 172
oversensitivity to smells 197

Oestradiol, menopausal hot flushes 156
Opium
adynamic/paralytic ileus 137
arousal after general anaesthesia 63
constipation 92
Oscillococcinum
bronchitis 79
common colds 90

Panax ginseng
postviral syndrome 179
weariness of mind 112
Perna canaliculus, bunions 80
Petroleum, motion sickness 159
Phosphorus
acute hepatitis 130
acute poststreptococcal glomerulonephritis 123
acute tracheitis 207
alcoholic neuritis 164
bad vibes, ill effects of 72
chronic pancreatitis 174
clairvoyance (excessive) 89
delirium tremens 98
dysentery 105
dyspareunia 105
Gilbert's syndrome 122
glaucoma (adjunctive therapy) 123
Grave's disease (adjunctive therapy) 125
haemorrhage 126
idiopathic thrombocytopenic purpura 183
laryngitis 148
pneumonia (adjunctive therapy) 178
rheumatoid arthritis 69
toning the voice 215
Phytolacca decandra
breast abscesses 78
fibrocystic breast disease 115
sore throats 197
Pitressin, acromegaly 57
Pituitarin, delayed puberty 183
Plantago, enuresis 110
Podophyllum
diarrhoea 102
rectal prolapse 181

Primula obconica, erythema
multiforme 111
Psorinum, offensive body odour 167
Pulsatilla
acute orchitis 169
amenorrhoea 62
arthritis 68, 69
breech presentation 78
bronchiectasis 79
brucellosis 80
catarrh 85
chronic sinusitis 196
cystic fibrosis 97
diarrhoea 101
epididymitis 110
galactorrhoea 121
German measles 122
gout 124
Grave's disease (adjunctive therapy)
125
hirsuitism, female 132
inadequate lactation 147
infantile fever 115
irritable bowel syndrome 143
measles 154
mumps 160
overindulgence 172
stys 200
Pulvis gunnorum
boils 77
incisional abscesses 56
Pyrogen, influenza 141

Ranunculus bulbosus
intercostal rheumatism 142
shingles 195
Rheum palmatum
diarrhoea 101
teething 203
Rhododendron, hydrocele 134
Rhus toxicodendron
ankylosing spondylitis 65
barber's itch 73
chickenpox 87
chilblains 87
ecthyma contagiosum 107
erythema nodosum 111
hand, foot and mouth disease 127
herpes simplex 131
lumbago 151
osteoarthritis 170
Reiter's syndrome 186
Sjögren's syndrome 196
Ruta graveolens
athletic support 70
eye strain 113
ganglia 121
post-extraction osteitis 104
repetitive strain injury 187
shin splints 194
sprains 198
tennis elbow 203
see also Injections: Ruta graveolens

Sabadilla, hay fever 128
Salix alba, lumbago 151
Sanguinaria, migraine 158
Secale, Raynaud's disease 185
Secretin, autism 71
Selenium
acne vulgaris 57
impotence 138
Senecio aureus, amenorrhoea 62
Sepia
alopecia 61
herpes simplex prevention 131
ovarian cysts, benign 96
postnatal depression 179
premenstrual syndrome 180
primary hypothyroidism 135
stress incontinence 199
uterine fibroids 116
uterine prolapse 181
Silicea
actinomycosis 58
athlete's foot 70
Bartholin's abscess and cyst 73
breast abscesses 78
bronchiectasis 79
catarrh 85
chalazion 85
chronic tonsillitis 207
cystic fibrosis 97
expulsion of embedded foreign
bodies 118
fistulae 117
glaucoma (adjunctive therapy)
123
hydrocele 134
lymphoedema of lower extremities
152
molluscum contagiosum 158
mucocele 160
osteomyelitis 170
otitis media 171
ovarian cysts, benign 96

paronychia 175
pilonidal sinus and abscess 177
Raynaud's disease 185
scabies 191
sinusitis 196
tonsillar hypertrophy 206
Sol, sunburn 200
Spigelia, migraine 158
Spongia tosta, croup 96
Staphisagria
analgesia 64
catheterization trauma 85
chalazion 85
cystitis 97
dyspareunia 105
irritability 143
love problems 150
psychological disorders following rape 185
sadism 190
sexual abuse 57
sexual frustration 194
stys 200
urethritis (adjunctive therapy) 210
vaginismus 212
Sticta pulmonaria, bursitis 81
Stramonium, delirium tremens 98
Streptococcinum, acute poststreptococcal glomerulonephritis 123
Sulphur
acromegaly 57
aphthous ulcers 67
Behçets disease 74
catarrh 85
enuresis 110
inappropriate sweating 210
offensive body odour 167
varicose eczema 213
Wegener's granulomatosis 216
Symphytum
black eye 76
osteogenesis imperfecta 170
to speed fracture union 119

Tabacum, motion sickness 159
Tarentula cubensis, carbuncles 83
Theridion, noise intolerance 165
Thiosinaminum
adhesions 58
frozen shoulder 195
scars 191
strictures 199
Thuja
antibiotics, ill effects of 65
chalazion 85
drug-induced rashes 104
immunization, prevention of adverse reactions 137
ranula 185
Thyroidinum
chronic urticaria 211
Grave's disease (adjunctive therapy) 125
primary hypothyroidism 135
Tilea europoea, chronic pelvic sepsis 176
Tuberculinum aviaire, acute bronchitis 79

Urtica urens
acute urticaria 211
solar urticaria 200

Viburnum opulus/prunifolium, abortion prevention 55
Vinca minor, alopecia 60

Zincum metallicum, restless leg syndrome 187

⁕ Bach Flower Remedies

Bach Agrimony
absenteeism 57
cheerfulness, deceptive 86, 145
desire for risky excitement 112, 189
drug addiction 58
easily manipulated persons 153
extroversion, deceptive 112
garrulousness 121
seekers of risky sex 194
seekers of wild distraction 175, 219
servility 193
show-offs 195
theatrical behaviour 204
unreliability 210
Bach Aspen
irrational fears 114, 132
terrifying dreams 104
Bach Beech
abruptness 56
aloofness 60
arrogance 68
bitchiness 75

Bach Beech (*cont.*)
bossiness 77
egotism 108
impatience 205
impudence/rudeness 138
indignation 139
intolerance 95, 128, 139, 142
irritability 143, 154
know-it-alls 146
nags 162
narrow-mindedness 163
obstinacy 167
ostracism 171
over-meticulousness 157, 176, 199
sanctimony 190
sarcasm 190
scepticism 191
snobbery 197
tendency to ridicule 189
vanity 213
Bach Centaury
drug addiction 58
easily manipulated persons 153
influence of others, ill effects of 140
lack of confidence 91
misguidedness 158
overwhelmed persons 172
overwork 173
slavish mothers 154
timidity 103
workaholism 217
Bach Cerato
advice-seeking, excessive 59
changeability 86
constant repetition 186
fickleness 116
greed for advice 125
indecisiveness 98
influence of others, ill effects of 140
loss of opportunities 168
misguidedness 158
need for reassurance 186
servility 193
unreliability 210
Bach Cherry Plum
fears for own sanity 190
hysteria 136
impetuosity 138
killers 146
nervous breakdowns 78
repetition of mistakes 186
ruthlessness 189
suicidal despair 100
uncontrollable laughter 148
violent fury 120
violent irritability 143
violent paranoia 174
violent rage 185
Bach Chestnut Bud
drug addiction withdrawal 58
failure to learn from mistakes 148, 158
Bach Chicory
argumentativeness 67
attention-seeking 137, 139
bitchiness 75
bitterness 76
bossiness 77
concern for others, excessive 91
craving for sympathy 201
delusions of grandeur 99
excessively house-proud persons 133
greed 125
impudence/rudeness 138
indignation 139
inquisitiveness 141
irritability 143
manipulative persons 153
meddlers 154
moodiness 159
nags 162
ostracism 171
over-strictness 199
possessiveness/selfishness 95, 114, 151, 154, 193
resentment 187
sarcasm 190
self-concern, excessive 91
sensitivity to criticism 95
show-offs 195
snobbery 197
sulks 200
theatrical behaviour 204
vanity 213
vindictiveness 214
Bach Clematis
absent-mindedness 57
absenteeism 57
apathy 66
boredom 77
carelessness 84
day-dreamers 220
feeling in a rut 189
inattentiveness 139
loners 150

love problems 150
procrastination 181
unpunctuality 205
unreliability 210
Bach Crab Apple
blemishes, preoccupation with 76
excessively house-proud persons 133
feeling ugly 209
feeling unclean 137, 185, 194
hypochondriasis 135
obsession with cosmetic surgery 93
obsessive hygiene/cleanliness 127, 134, 176, 177
over-meticulousness 157
self-disgust 92, 95, 102
sexual abuse 57
shame, excessive 194
Bach Elm
absenteeism 57
easily discouraged persons 102
failure to cope 114
malingerers 153
overburden 81
too much responsibility 172, 187
Bach Gentian
easily discouraged persons 59, 102, 169, 194
lack of confidence 91
negative personalities 102
Bach Gorse
convalescence 93
excessive scepticism 191
hopelessness of the sick 59, 90
pessimism 133, 194
resignation to ill-health 187, 189
Bach Heather
cravings for sympathy 201
garrulousness 121, 175, 186
need for company 125, 144
obsession with symptoms/ailments 111, 135, 137
obsession with youthfulness 219
ostracism 171
self-concern, excessive 91
selfishness 193
Bach Holly
bitchiness 75
distrust 103
embitterment 76, 109
envy 110
flippancy 117
fury 120
hatred 109, 128, 139
hoarding 133
irritability 143
jealousy 145
killers 146
lack of sympathy 201
mercilessness 157
ostracism 171
paranoia 174
passionate and jealous love 150
rage 185
resentment 187, 188
revenge 188
ruthlessness 189
sadism 190
sarcasm 190
scepticism 191
tendency to ridicule 189
theatrical behaviour 204
unrequited love 151
vindictiveness 214
worrying thoughts 204
Bach Honeysuckle
bereavement 74
constant reminiscence 175, 186, 188
distraction by memories 103, 139
dwelling upon past love 150
homesickness 133
poor memory 155
regrets 186
unpleasant memories 165, 204
Bach Hornbeam
apathy 66
convalescence 93
drug addiction withdrawal 58
fatigue from sexual overindulgence 194
mental exhaustion 112
Monday morning syndrome 158
morning-after feeling 220
procrastination 181
Bach Impatiens
abruptness 56
argumentativeness 67
boredom 77
bossiness 77
carelessness 84
constant repetition 186
distraction 103
excess haste 134
flippancy 117
garrulousness 121

Bach Impatiens (*cont.*)
impatience 132, 137, 139, 205
impetuosity 138
inability to delegate 98
inquisitiveness, excessive 141
intolerance 142
irritability 143
isolation 144
keenness, excessive 146
loners 150
meddling 154
mistakes, from rushing 158
overwhelmed persons 172
rage 185
sex, over too quickly 194
tongue-tied persons 206
Bach Larch
avoidance of responsibility 187
doubts about sexual competence 194
expectation of failure 114
lack of confidence 91, 169, 206
need for reassurance 186
procrastination 181
Bach Mimulus
fear of abandonment 55
fear of the consequences of sex 194
fear of failure 114
fear of growing old 219
fear of illness 137
hoarders 133
lack of confidence 91
need for reassurance 186
procrastination 181
rational fears 114
tongue-tied persons 206
unreliability 210
vaginismus 212
Bach Mustard, convalescence 93
Bach Oak
concern for others, excessive 91, 114
exaggerated sense of duty 104
frustration due to illness 137
inability to delegate 98
overwork 81, 173, 217
soldiering on 59, 187, 194
Bach Olive
absent-mindedness 57
carelessness 84
convalescence 93
exhaustion 112, 153, 173
Bach Pine
feelings of failure 114
guilt 95, 185, 194
over-apologetic persons 67, 166
premature ejaculation 180
regrets 186
self-blame 158
self-contempt 92
servility 193
sexual abuse 57
Bach Red Chestnut
fears for others 91, 114, 140
overly unselfish mothers 154
Bach Rescue Remedy
collapse 90
fright 119
hysteria 136
terrifying dreams 104
terror 203
Bach Rock Rose
nightmares following rape 185
terrifying dreams 104
terror of growing old 219
Bach Rock Water
delusions of grandeur 99
exaggerated sense of duty 105
fitness freaks 219
hoarders 133
intolerance 142
isolation 144
martyrdom 154
narrow-mindedness 163
over-meticulousness 157
over-strictness about self 102, 188, 199
sadism 190
sanctimony 190
self-perfectionism 91, 95, 132, 133, 157, 176
snobbery 197
time-specific rituals 205
vanity 213
workaholism 217
zealotry 220
Bach Scleranthus
confused sexuality 194
fickleness 86, 116
indecisiveness 98, 103, 181
lost opportunities 168
mood swings 159
unreliability 210
Bach Star of Bethlehem
bad news 72
bereavement 74
psychological shock 185, 220

Bach Sweet Chestnut, despair 100, 133
Bach Vervain
  altruism, ill effects of 61
  argumentativeness 67
  bossiness 77
  concern for others, excessive 91
  constant repetition 186
  criticism of others 95
  delusions of grandeur 99
  difficulty retiring 188
  driven persons 205
  egotism 108
  enjoyment of confrontation 91
  enthusiasm, excessive 109, 146
  exaggerated sense of duty 104
  excitement by risks 189
  fury at injustices 120
  fussiness 157
  garrulousness 121
  highly strung persons 132
  impetuosity 138
  inability to delegate 98
  indignation 139
  inquisitiveness, excessive 141
  intolerance 142
  irritability 143
  martyrdom 154
  meddling 154
  obstinacy 167
  overexcitement by sexual images 194
  overwork 81, 173
  poor memory 155
  rage 185
  resentment 187
  sanctimony 190
  sensitivity to criticism 95
  show-offs 195
  strictness 199
  theatrical behaviour 154, 204
  tongue-tied persons 206
  workaholism 217
  zealotry 220
Bach Vine
  abruptness 56
  aloofness 60
  arrogance 68, 184
  bossiness 77, 102
  enjoyment of confrontation 91
  fury 120
  inability to delegate 98
  irritability 143
  know-it-alls 146
  merciless dictators 157
  nags 162
  obstinacy 167
  power freaks 95, 108, 125, 139, 176
  rage 185
  ruthlessness 189
  sadism 190
  sanctimony 190
  sarcasm 190
  scepticism 191
  selfishness 193
  sensitivity to criticism 95
  sexual dominance, excessive 194
  show-offs 195
  snobbery 197
  tendency to ridicule 189
  tyranny 199
  unsympathetic persons 210
  vindictiveness 214
Bach Walnut
  adaptation to retirement 188
  bad vibes 72
  changes, ill effects of 86
  cutting ties with past 168, 175
  drug addiction withdrawal 58
  influence of others, ill effects of 140
  lack of confidence 91
  misguided persons 158
  regrets 186
Bach Water Violet
  aloofness 60
  dislike of sex 194
  isolation 144
  loners 150
Bach White Chestnut
  distraction by worries 103
  inattentiveness 139
  poor memory 155
  victim's preoccupation with rape 185
  worrying thoughts 204
Bach Wild Oat
  boredom 77
  feeling in a rut 189
  fickleness 116
  indecisiveness 98
  loss of opportunities 168
  need for reassurance 186
  uncertainty about future 175, 188
Bach Wild Rose
  apathy 66, 194, 220
  dispassionateness 103

Bach Wild Rose (*cont.*)
malingering 153
procrastination 181
resignation 187, 188, 189
unpunctuality 205
Bach Willow
argumentativeness 67
craving sympathy 210
embitterment 76, 109
envy 110
grumbling 187
hatred 128
impudence/rudeness 138
irritability 143
moodiness 159
ostracism 171
resentment of illness 90
sarcasm 190
self-pity and resentment 91
selfishness 193
sensitivity to criticism 95
sulks 200

Injections

Hydroxocobalamin *see* Vitamin B12

Ruta graveolens
carpal tunnel syndrome 84
coccidynia 89
frozen shoulder 195
lumbago 151
muscular/ligamentous strain 199
Osgood-Schlatter's disease 169
osteoarthritis 170
repetitive strain injury 187
sciatica 192
sprains 198
tennis elbow 203

Vitamin B12 (hydroxocobalamin)
Alzheimer's disease 62
Bell's palsy 74
burning foot syndrome 81
burning mouth syndrome 81
bursitis 81
chronic urticaria 211
eczema, internal therapy 107
erythema multiforme 111
giardiasis 122
glandular fever 123
idiopathic vitiligo 215
male infertility 140
neuralgia 164
postviral syndrome 179
premenstrual syndrome 180
shingles 195
tinnitus 205

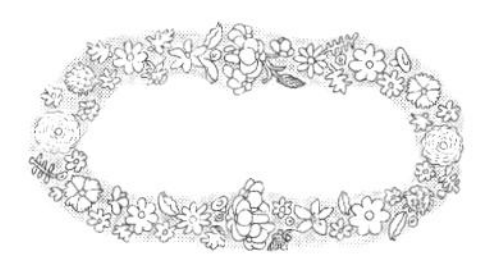